Advance praise for
Predictive Health

"Medicine is undergoing a transformation from being reactive to disease events to being predictive, preventive, and personalized. In *Predictive Health*, two leaders of the emerging field of predictive health care give readers an informative and interesting view of this health revolution and what it means to them."

—Ralph Snyderman, M.D., Chancellor Emeritus,
Duke University, and past CEO/President,
Duke University Health System

"This is a book everyone should read—not just scientists, ethicists, and those interested in the health of our people, but the public. The authors get it: the goal is to have early old age last as long as possible and late old age last 15 minutes. They give us ways to get there that are visionary today, and will be proven to have been prophetic 30 years from now."

—Arthur Garson, Jr., M.D., M.P.H., Director,
Center for Health Policy, University of Virginia,
and coauthor of *Health Care Half Truths*

"*Predictive Health* is a refreshing read—it looks at medicine in a whole new light. Instead of focusing on disease, the authors explore new ways to think about our own health. They weave together basic and applied science—including the human genome and its impact—in an understandable way. Above all, their main message is that life and death are intertwined and we humans need to learn to deal with that concept as we go through life."

—Edward D. Miller, M.D.,
Dean/CEO Emeritus, Johns Hopkins Medicine

Predictive Health

Predictive Health

HOW WE CAN REINVENT MEDICINE TO EXTEND OUR BEST YEARS

Kenneth Brigham, M.D.

AND

Michael M. E. Johns, M.D.

BASIC BOOKS

A Member of the Perseus Books Group
New York

Published by Basic Books,
A Member of the Perseus Books Group

Books published by Basic Books are available at special discounts for
bulk purchases in the United States by corporations, institutions, and
other organizations. For more information, please contact the Special
Markets Department at the Perseus Books Group, 2300 Chestnut Street,
Suite 200, Philadelphia, PA 19103, or call (800) 810-4145, ext. 5000,
or e-mail special.markets@perseusbooks.com.

Designed by Brent Wilcox

A CIP catalog record for this book is available from
the Library of Congress.
Hardcover ISBN: 978-0-465-02312-7
E-book ISBN: 978-0-465-03299-0

10 9 8 7 6 5 4 3 2 1

To our wives,
Arlene Stecenko and Trina Johns

Contents

Contents

Authors' Note

Several years ago, Emory University engaged in a broad exploration of the future of biomedicine in America that resulted in the adoption of "Predictive Health and Society" as a transdisciplinary and transinstitutional strategic theme. This book grew from our participation in and interpretation of that process. We won't incriminate the large group of involved faculty from Emory University, the Georgia Institute of Technology, and the Centers for Disease Control and Prevention by mentioning their names; we have drawn our own conclusions from their deliberations and accept full responsibility for what we have written. This book also draws on a body of research and other information found in published books and articles and at many Internet sites. We do not include specific references and footnotes in the text in order to make the book more readable, but at the end of the book there is for each chapter a list of sources and additional reading, mostly including material written for a general audience. Finally, we have drawn from our own personal experience in biomedicine as educators, investigators, practitioners, and administrators, encompassing, between us, almost a century. Hilda Echt and Carleton Hensley, to whom we refer throughout the book, were real people, and the descriptions of them are as accurate as memory permits, but we have changed their names to respect their memories. Although we have attempted to verify facts, there are undoubtedly errors, and they are our fault; we apologize in advance to the reader.

We thank Jennifer Vazquez and Lynn Cunningham for their invaluable help in evolving the concept of Predictive Health and for their support with the logistics of producing this book. We also thank Anita Bray, Ashley Teal, and the staff of the Emory Georgia Tech Center for Health Discovery and Well Being® for the many things they do that made the book possible. Our agent, Diane Freed with FinePrint Literary Agency, is responsible for finding a comfortable home for the work with Basic Books; we very much appreciate her efforts. The book is much improved by the diligent efforts of T. J. Kelleher, our editor at Basic Books.

Predictive Health

PART I

The Challenge and the Opportunity

As many of us as possible should age with grace and die with painless dignity of natural causes.

CHAPTER 1

Ponce's Dream

EVEN HAD THE sixteenth-century explorer Juan Ponce de León found the fabled fountain of youth, it may not have saved him from the fatal consequences of the Native American's arrow that found its mark during his second and final visit to the land he called Pascua de Florida. The compelling thing about his quest is that he risked his life chasing so wispy a rumor. But then the vision of perpetual, even apparent, health is a potent motivator; ask any plastic surgeon or cosmetic manufacturer.

The promise of at least prolonged, if not perpetual, health no longer rests on rumor. Existing and emerging science and technology give substance to the hope, even the expectation, that we can understand enough about health and how to keep it to let us live longer and better than we could have imagined even a decade ago. That knowledge and how to deal with it is what we call Predictive Health, defining what health is and detecting and correcting the earliest unhealthy tendencies long before there is any evidence of disease. The challenge of translating that knowledge into practice involves more than science and technology. Realizing the possibilities will require major changes in how human beings—scientists, health practitioners, and politicians, as well as people in general—think and behave. We can have health care—predictive health care—that is accessible, affordable, humane, ethical, and efficient. We can do it, if only we can figure out how.

Biomedicine in the United States is largely focused on disease; that is, organ failure. We spend most of our resources—money and people—in both biomedical research and clinical care on understanding and treating disease, even though disease is a very late consequence of long malfunctioning processes and is often irreversible. Research with this focus births dramatic (and expensive) interventions that too often have less than optimal effects on quality of life. Fully a third of the national Medicare budget is spent in the final year of life, and a third of that amount is spent in the last month of life, often on expensive and futile treatments in intensive care units. This arrangement is not sustainable. We may have the best disease care system in the world, but we do not have the best health-care system.

Health has been defined traditionally as the absence of disease, a definition without much utility in a health-focused system (theoretically, to declare a person healthy it would be necessary to rule out every possible disease, at best an impractical effort). Social need, cost, and fundamental discoveries will force major changes in health care, shifting the goal from treating disease to maintaining health. New programs of this sort with novel titles are already appearing at major academic institutions and health-care companies. That shift should gather momentum as the tools for measuring health and predicting disease proliferate and improved efficiency and cost/benefit ratios become more apparent.

The shift in focus of biomedical research has been slower to develop. We need to focus the formidable power of the research enterprise—basic, translational, and clinical—on developing a positive definition of health in quantitative terms. This would provide powerful new tools for health surveillance, assessing risk, and premorbid diagnosis, as well as rationales for new interventions at early stages of unhealth that would preclude progression to overt disease.

Driving this new paradigm for health care are the rapidly advancing fields of genomics and proteomics. Lee Hood, founder of the Institute for Systems Biology in Seattle, predicts that the technology for genome sequencing (genomics) and measuring serum concentrations of a thousand or more proteins (proteomics) will be easy and cheap enough to be applied to individual health care within a decade or so. Other technologies, including nanotechnology and molecular imaging, could add detail to characterizing health, further enhancing the ability to measure health and detect tendencies to develop disease.

Not long ago, within the lifetime of many of us still practicing medicine, a dominant ethic held that death was a medical failure. Everything possible was done to keep people technically alive—to prolong the agonal gasp. In this more enlightened time, doctors have more respect for the inevitability of death and feel obliged to dignify that event as much as possible, but death is still the enemy to be conquered. In the new paradigm, it is disease, not death, that will be the medical failure.

The ease with which data are gathered is changing the landscape, enabled by the discipline of bioinformatics. Masses of information about the most intimate molecular events essential to life and health come from a drop of blood or the few cells dislodged from the inside of a cheek by the gentle scrape of a cotton swab. The irrepressible urge of scientists to classify and categorize information has added the suffix "ome" to descriptors of life processes: genome, epigenome, transcriptome, proteome, metabolome, even interactome. Such labels make scientists feel better about bodies of information too big and complex for the unaided human brain to fathom.

Fortunately the creativity of the human brain has let us make an electronic end run around that complexity. Computer power can domesticate the "omes" into tractable knowledge that is comprehensible to mortals and yields rationales for constructive action. Not only will we understand life processes at a level beyond what we can now imagine, but we will learn how to influence those processes to keep them working right—data, evidence, and hard facts will ultimately trump intuition.

Technologies developing at near-breakneck speed are continually increasing the possibilities. Nanotechnology is an example. Machines the size of a molecule could be manufactured and engineered to sense events in cells and alter them in specific ways that encourage normal functions. These "nanoparticles" (including one breed dubbed "quantum dots") could be injected into a vein, targeted to specific cells, and have their behavior and actions tracked by special detectors outside the body, providing incredibly detailed and precise data, collected with minimal violation of one's person.

Emerging generations of devices integrated with sophisticated electronics can produce exquisite images of organs (and before long, even individual cells) without so much as touching the imagee. Holographic displays of those images are eerily realistic. The most arcane of anatomical crannies could be examined in astounding detail while avoiding the discomfort and humiliation imposed by the proliferating number of medical scopes.

Numerous other technologies will make it possible to define health and detect the earliest unhealthy tendencies. This very personal information will identify new targets for intervention and provide the means for tracking the results. This is individual, personalized health care. Testing new treatments will not depend on statistical evaluations in large groups. Effects will be measured in each person, and conclusions about treatments will be just as specific.

However, science and technology will only provide some tools. Turning these advances into a health-care system will force us to reckon with ethical, social, behavioral, economic, political, legal, and commercial issues that science alone will not solve. Advances in each of those areas should proceed in parallel with scientific developments, informed by rich transdisciplinary dialogue. Communication among a broad spectrum of disciplines will happen only if scholars, investigators, and practitioners have both the motive and the opportunity to interact.

The cold fact is that the system will follow the money. What will be done—what research and what health care—will be what the people footing the bill (mostly governments and insurance companies) decide to pay for. Although a unique convergence of science, technology, and social milieu can make the change possible, the economics are complex, and the implications of change are threatening. The decision makers will have to muster the will and good sense to make it happen. There is a window of opportunity, but it may not be large.

Predictive Health will not realize Ponce de León's dream. It will not confer immortality or eternal youth, but it could make mortal events a brief and amiable consequence of the human organism having exhausted its natural span of life. Too many of us—like Carleton Hensley, a Baltimore steelworker who will accompany us throughout this book—live long enough to retire from a grueling job but not much longer. Too few of us—like Hilda Echt, an affluent Atlantan—thrive for a century despite occasional physical challenges. In the contrasting experiences of these two real people we will find, if not a path to the fountain of youth, then maybe something better. As many of us as possible should age with grace and die with painless dignity of natural causes. How can we do that?

CHAPTER 2

Disease as a Medical Failure

A Transforming Paradigm

SOMETIME IN THE early hours of July 1, 1966, Carleton Hensley, a retired Sparrow's Point welder, was admitted from the
Johns Hopkins Hospital accident room to an acute unit of the hospital's charity wing. Mr. Hensley was incoherent, his diabetes de-
compensated, his long-abused liver and ailing kidneys failing, taxed
past their limits. Barely past its sixtieth year, his body was already
used up, exhausted by excess, neglect, and bad choices.

In 1966, even at the elite Johns Hopkins Hospital in Baltimore,
there were no intensive care units. On Osler 2—the second floor of
the charity service's acute wing, named for William Osler, the near-
mythical godfather of modern American medicine—there was one
four-bed ward with window air conditioners that was reserved for
victims of heart attacks. Mr. Hensley and the other patients on
Osler 2 lay nearly naked in pools of sweat in the searing summer
heat. Mr. Hensley's failing body generated more heat, a side effect of
the desperate metabolic burst typical of the failing human organism. The heat encased him, driving his core temperature into the
red zone.

Early that morning a young M.D., freshly graduated near the
top of his class from one of the most distinguished American medical schools, lay awake, anxiously awaiting the phone call that would

announce his first admission as an intern. He had competed successfully for one of the very best medical residencies in the world and trembled with the adrenalin rush, anticipating his first experience as a real doctor, the chance to save a human life. Wasn't saving lives what it was about? That's how success was measured. Death was a medical failure, and so a doctor's failure. Internalizing that ethos had propelled him to the top of his class and given him the sacred opportunity to be a player in the life-and-death games of serious human illness. That opportunity would happen at the intersection of his and Mr. Hensley's paths.

One of the first classic emergencies that one learns about in medical school is diabetic ketoacidosis (DKA). There is a formula for treating it. There are unambiguous signals from blood and urine measurements that tell how a patient is responding. Mr. Hensley appeared to be a straightforward case of the disorder. The young intern wrote his orders with confidence and read the test results with satisfaction. Mr. Hensley was responding well.

But there was more. When the intern held his patient's wrist and extended his patient's hand, the hand flapped up and down—asterixis, a telltale sign of liver failure. And his eyes were yellow, clearly yellow now. That wasn't mentioned in the accident room note. His temperature, too, continued to rise; there had to be infection somewhere, although his urine was clear and the chest X-ray was okay. Need an x-ray of his abdomen. Peritonitis? Retroperitoneal abscess? Something in there that cannot be seen or felt with unaided human senses.

The X-ray helped—a subtle sign of retroperitoneal abscess, a pocket of pus trapped along the inside of the back muscles. Like a boil, it had to be drained for the infection to clear.

The surgical chief resident didn't want to touch Mr. Hensley—the man was a train wreck, he said. No sense in doing surgery; too many things were wrong. It was too big a risk. But the patient was sure to die otherwise, and the intern's argument prevailed, the surgeon responding to the desperation in the intern's voice. We can't just let him die; we have to do something, anything, that has a chance of working.

So the surgery was done and the abscess drained.

It wasn't enough. Mr. Hensley subsequently developed several other sites of infection, his enfeebled diabetic immune system too weak to maintain the barrier between him and the vast microbial world. After a week's stormy hospitalization, during which he regained enough coherence to recognize his devoted wife, who did not leave his side—grasping her hand, clinging with what strength he could muster to his rapidly waning shard of life—Mr. Hensley died.

The intern sat with Mrs. Hensley in the waiting room, both of them exhausted from the ordeal, and they cried together. She had lost her most valued companion for the past thirty years, the love of her life. He had lost a battle to save a life, a battle critical to his image of himself as a doctor. The war was not lost, but his confidence was shaken. Medicine had failed. He had failed. He was unaccustomed to failure.

Medicine has entered another millennium since 1966, both literally and figuratively. There have been (and continue to be) enormous technological developments, masses of new knowledge for understanding disease and treating failing organs. But medicine is still obsessed with prolonging life at all costs. The same ethos that guided Mr. Hensley's treatment is responsible for a large portion of the dollars spent on health care in the United States (e.g., organ transplantation, dialysis, elaborate life support in intensive care units), an amount totaling more than 17 percent of the gross domestic product and growing fast. We have developed an elaborate and envied disease care system. If we contract a serious disease, we want to be treated in the United States.

But if we were British, and without a terminal disease, we could expect to live five years longer than we will as Americans, even though the British spend half as much per person per year on health care as Americans do. In fact, life expectancy in the United States is markedly shorter than it is in virtually every other developed country, even though the United States far outstrips all of those countries in health-care spending as a fraction of the wealth each country generates.

Our experience—we are both well-to-do physicians with stable jobs and solid insurance—is not like that of many Americans, upwards of fifty million of whom have no health insurance. Like Mr. Hensley, they have access to the medical system only when they are already desperately ill. The uninsured do not have the luxury of choosing preventive care, or having their chronic disease diagnosed early and given careful attention, limiting painful and expensive complications. Their primary doctor is in the emergency room where the bleeding is staunched, bone set, metabolism put minimally back on track for a few hours, long enough to get them out the door upright and conscious. They don't get serious and prolonged attention without the catastrophic failure of something . . . or everything.

It is catastrophic failure that fuels the system. Medical schools train doctors to diagnose and treat disease. People who see doctors are considered patients—illness is assumed; it's just a matter of giving it a name, making the diagnosis. Both the intellectual and technical satisfaction that health-care providers derive from practicing medicine depends on disease . . . organ failure . . . biological catastrophe. Practitioners of any profession do what they are trained to do, behave as they have learned to behave. Doctors trained to focus their efforts on and derive both their livelihood and their personal satisfaction from diagnosing and treating disease will do just that, and do it with rapidly increasing technological sophistication, regardless of an even more rapidly increasing cost. That is the dogma we perpetuate.

The cost of Carleton Hensley's terminal illness in 1966 was a week's hospitalization, several batteries of blood tests, and an operation. The intern who was his primary doctor and the surgical resident who did the operation were paid by the system as part of their training. Because Mr. Hensley was cared for in a charity ward, Mrs. Hensley may not have received a bill from the Johns Hopkins Hospital. If she did, it is virtually certain that no effort was made to collect. The system did not compound biological and emotional catastrophe with financial ruin.

A Mr. Hensley in this millennium would almost certainly live longer than he did in 1966. He would be rushed in an express elevator from the emergency room to a gleaming heat- and humidity-regulated, intensive-care biosphere. He would have tubes inserted into numerous natural and created orifices. His body would be attached to a battery of machines, some to do what he could not do for himself, some to measure and display what was happening in living color on flat-screen plasma television. There would be CAT scans, MRIs, maybe even PET scans. Maybe renal dialysis in a desperate attempt to filter out the toxins, to abort the inevitable course of things. A senior attending critical care physician would keep careful tabs on the fledgling interns and residents, countersigning notes in the chart, checking orders, making sure that the residents did not spend more than the designated eighty hours per week on the unit—there are billing and accreditation to worry about, requirements to make sure the hospital is playing strictly by the rules.

A twenty-first-century Mr. Hensley would surely live longer, but not much longer. He would have at most a few more weeks of life, the bulk of it spent as an appendage of the technology, in a fog of sedatives and analgesics with a tube in his throat, pulsating with each thrust of the ventilator. He would be unable to communicate. After some weeks of this, when the futility became impossible to ignore, there would be a family conference. Mrs. Hensley would have to decide to pull the plug, stop the futile heroics. The decision would not be easy; Mrs. Hensley would cry. The two residents who would present the options, dry eyed, to Mrs. Hensley would have been "on the case" only a couple of days. And Mrs. Hensley would certainly get bills. An average day in a modern intensive care unit (ICU) costs upward of $10,000. Multiply that by twenty or thirty and add all the other costs. A retired Sparrows Point welder's entire net worth might not approach that bottom line. Medicare would help, and there might be some other sources, but the cost to the system would be enormous. And what did it buy?

If our twenty-first-century Mr. Hensley were fortunate enough to have private insurance, it might well have covered most of the costs of his final illness. What it almost certainly would not have paid for is the kind of attentive care for his diabetes, given long before his final visit to the emergency room, that could have prolonged his healthier life, at least forestalling the final catastrophe and possibly preventing it altogether. The system, the entire system, is driven by catastrophe. Something serious has to fail before the system responds.

The system will change because it must. We will not tolerate forever a health-care system that costs too much and delivers too little. Quality and access are just part of the problem. Continually escalating cost, unchecked, will drive the current system out of business.

The system will also change because it can. We live in a vortex of discovery and invention that is spinning out at a dizzying pace new tools for measuring health. We already have much of the technology for predicting an individual person's health and measuring the consequences of healthy (or unhealthy) living. And it is difficult to imagine the possibilities a decade or two from now.

Inevitable change is unique opportunity. Imagine a healthy infant Carleton Hensley born in the middle of the twenty-first century. A drop of blood from a tiny heel prick, barely noticed in the squalling bustle of the birth scene, passed through a maze of tiny automatic analyzers, yields information, thousands of bits of information, to a database, where the bits are assembled into a picture of health, Carleton Hensley's health, now and in the future. He's at risk for type II diabetes and may have trouble controlling his appetites on occasion; he should probably be educated pretty aggressively about alcohol and drugs as he grows up and is tempted; and a lot of attention should be paid to his diet, starting now. A doctor (or maybe some new breed of health-care professional) will partner with Carleton's parents to outline a lifelong health plan for the child. They will make arrangements to keep in touch, via the Web, telephone, personal visits. They will be partners. This is commitment.

Mr. Carleton Hensley will enter the twenty-second millennium in robust health, continuing to work and pay taxes. His only reason for contact with a hospital in eighty-five years of life will be a broken arm from a bicycle accident, set in an emergency room and healed uneventfully. At a ripe old age, having used up his allotted time, he will die at home surrounded by a caring family. And the cost for Mr. Hensley's lifelong health care will have been less than the cost of a monthlong stay in an early twenty-first-century ICU. Add the value of several more years of productive life, and the economics start to get pretty compelling. The human value is even more compelling.

Care focused on health instead of exclusively on disease could have meant that Mr. Hensley would have lived longer and healthier. Keeping him from developing diabetes and helping him control some unhealthy urges speaks to his biology, his physical health. But human beings are more beautifully complex than is apparent from their biology alone. Physical problems may be symptoms of deeper phenomena. There is reason to think that we can understand more of that complexity and that it will make a difference in how healthy people are. Could that understanding have meant that Mr. Hensley would have thrived for a century, completely free of diabetes and the other problems he faced? Maybe. Then again, maybe not. Try as we might, some things that affect individual health and longevity may remain beyond our reach.

CHAPTER 3

Toward Exemplary Health

HILDA ECHT WAS one hundred years old when she invited a stranger to lunch at her upscale Atlanta retirement home. She had rehabilitated from a stroke and survived uterine cancer a few years earlier. Her bones, having done their job for all those years, now couldn't support even her ninety-pound frame without the help of a walker. But she met her guest at the door and guided him to the large dining room.

There was still a hint of what must have been a spring in her now-halting step. She spoke to everyone she passed, asking about their welfare in a strong lilting voice and elaborating the details of their various challenges sotto voce to her guest. Her expression was fixed in a warm smile, and her eyes were bright. She occasionally laughed a small, private laugh, as though there were a cache of amusements stored away in that venerable brain that continued to entertain her.

"What do you think is the thing old people need the most?" she asked, challenging her doctor guest from a position of clearly superior knowledge of the needs of the aged.

"Medical care," was his stock answer.

"Hogwash," she replied. "If you get to be as old as I am, you get medical care. Otherwise you'd have died off a long time ago. It's transportation. Getting places just to do the essentials is a problem, much less getting out and among people. I drove until I was past ninety. Without that car, I'm grounded like a naughty teenager."

Seated at her regular table, Ms. Echt and her guest scanned the dining room. Men and women with varying degrees of mobility milled about a lunch buffet. Many spoke to Ms. Echt or waved at her, mouthing a greeting. A waiter came to the table, greeted her, and handed her guest a menu.

"Your usual lunch, Ms. Echt?" the waiter asked.

"Yes, Herman," she answered. "And how are you today?"

"Fine, thank you. And you have yet another guest today, I see," he said.

The two-hour lunch that followed was a crash course in geriatrics for Ms. Echt's guest, and he never forgot the lesson. He was especially struck by what seemed to him the dominant feature of this hundred-year-old woman's personality. She was connected, deliberately and aggressively connected, to other people. Was she healthy? Well, she was alive and had lived productively for a century. She had raised and educated her children, escorting them into successful professional careers and seeing them through to retirement. She had obtained a master's degree at seventy and started a philanthropic foundation. She had self-published a number of small books dealing with the needs of old people and approaches to their care and support. Hard to argue with that, even if atherosclerosis and cancer had taken shots at her and she needed a walker.

When the conversation turned to death and dying, Ms. Echt said, "I want to drop dead . . . but not yet." She died two years later. Maybe she was ready by then.

The big challenge facing us is how to redesign health care so that the Mr. Hensleys of the world also have the chance to live a full and good life until they are ready to die. We made the point previously that the way this country is doing health care now—focusing on disease instead of health and viewing death as the enemy to be conquered—isn't doing that. Ms. Echt's story is a good place to start developing that idea.

This country's approach to understanding human health has parallels in the apocryphal parable of the six blind men and the elephant. Each man firmly concluded that an elephant was like a wall, a snake, a spear, a tree, a fan, or a rope, depending on whether the part he felt was the side, the trunk, the tusk, the leg, the ear, or the tail. The original story is from the Buddhist tradition, but John Godfrey Saxe translated its essence into a deceptively amusing poem, called appropriately, "The Blind Men and the Elephant." Although he was commenting on the nature of theological discussions of his time, the final two stanzas of his poem are equally valid for present-day medicine:

And so these men of Indostan, disputed loud and long,
each in his own opinion, exceeding stiff and strong,
Though each was partly in the right, and all were in the wrong!

So, oft in theologic wars, the disputants, I ween,
tread on in utter ignorance, of what each other mean,
and prate about the elephant, not one of them has seen!

Most doctors, like that Hopkins intern in 1966 who pressed desperate interventions on a dying Carleton Hensley, mistake the part of the medical story that we know best for the whole picture. However, as long ago as 1948 the World Health Organization (WHO) defined health as "a state of complete physical, mental and social well-being and not merely the absence of disease or infirmity." So some people caught a glimpse of the whole elephant over half a century ago, at least in theory. But medicine, both before and since 1948 (at least from the early twentieth century, when the Flexner report ushered in the modern medical era), has pretty much limited itself to the biology (the physical part), defying WHO and defining health precisely as "the absence of disease or infirmity."

The benefits of that approach have been remarkable. Modern medicine has cured a number of diseases and controlled others. We don't live in fear of a plague epidemic. Development and extensive use of vaccines have almost eliminated smallpox and dramatically reduced the incidence of a host of viral illnesses (including polio) that were once major threats. Antibiotics have robbed many malignant bacteria of their power to maim and kill. Cancer is an obstinate and resourceful foe, but advances in surgical technique and chemotherapy have made inroads there as well. Devices can be implanted to rescue a quivering heart or boost a failing one. Healthy organs—hearts, lungs, livers, kidneys, pancreases—can be transplanted from donors to recipients whose organs have failed. These miracles of modern medicine are the product of a laserlike focus on disease as the target, with health perceived as what's left after disease is ruled out or cured.

Others have concerned themselves with "physical, mental and social well-being." Psychologists, sociologists, theologians, adherents of what is commonly called "holistic" health, and humanists in general have explored the concept of well-being and how emotions, social experience, and other behavioral and environmental factors affect it. As with the physical focus of medicine, major advances have been made. We (the royal we) understand better than ever many facets of human experience, but each area of understanding is packaged in a distinct parcel and guarded behind rigid boundaries of vocabulary, mindset, disciplinary bias, and territorial jealousy.

Given how we have chosen to organize information (and education) and the escalating complexity of crossing disciplinary boundaries, territorial behavior is inevitable; it is the nature of the beast. And though disciplines are convenient ways to organize things, their boundaries are artificial and arbitrary. The more we learn, the more

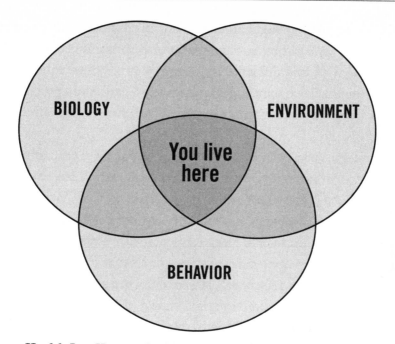

Health Is a Human Condition, Not Just a Biological Fact

obvious that becomes. Meanwhile, we are content to "prate about the elephant not one of [us] has seen," satisfied with being partly right but completely wrong. The result is that we know how to "create" a Carleton Hensley but not a Hilda Echt. There is a moral imperative to change that.

The figure above is a simple attempt at visualizing relationships among major influences on health presented as a Venn diagram. One major influence is biology, some of which we can't do anything about (like genetic predilections or some forms of cancer). But environment and behavior in their broadest sense also have major influences on health and well-being. And the reality is that we live in the middle of the figure, in the space where biology, behavior, and environment overlap, each affecting the other in a cloud of resonating signals. The bad news is that we don't know much about how to change a Carleton Hensley's fundamental biology. The good news is that his behavior and environment could be controlled in ways that influence his biology for the better. Hilda Echt may have had some advantageous fundamental biology, but her good fortune was no doubt also a result of how she behaved and where she lived.

An increasing body of science demonstrates the clear interdependence of biology, environment, and behavior. A few examples illustrate the point.

One study compared the immune systems of people enduring the chronic stress of caring for loved ones with Alzheimer's disease to those of otherwise similar people without that stress. Unsurprisingly, chronically stressed people were more depressed. But detailed tests of the health of immune cells known as lymphocytes showed that the stressed people's immune systems, the principal guardians of the physically healthy state, were compromised. More than that, the stressed peoples' lymphocytes had short telomeres. Telomeres are little snippets of DNA that are essential for cells to replicate, and they get shorter as we get older. Eventually they are so short that cells can't divide anymore, a condition we call senility. These essential immune cells in the stressed people were prematurely old and dysfunctional. Social/emotional experiences and physical phenomena do not occur independently. We live in the middle of the Venn diagram.

Two psychiatrists, Miller and Raison, noticed that people given interferon-α as treatment for cancer often became depressed. The human body produces interferon-α as part of a response to foreign invaders, called inflammation. Since provoking inflammation causes depression, these psychiatrists wondered whether the opposite was true, whether depression triggers inflammation (it does). Amounts of several chemicals that indicate inflammation were higher in the blood of people who were depressed, regardless of the cause.

Even early life experiences can affect how the body responds to stress later in life. For example, depressed adult men who have experienced some kind of increased stress in their childhood have an exaggerated inflammatory response to psychosocial stress. Perhaps there is even a third dimension to the Venn diagram: time. A cumulative interaction of biology, environment, and behavior may determine how healthy (or unhealthy) each of us is over the long haul.

Experiences can also favor health. Aging women who, like Ms. Echt, are engaged in self-development and personal growth, sleep better and have lower amounts of inflammatory chemicals in their blood than their less-engaged peers. Health must be viewed in the context of the larger human experience—the human condition is not simply a biological fact.

The passive definition of health as the absence of disease and the perception of health as a purely physical phenomenon were useful in an earlier time, when medicine was largely empirical and diagnostic technology sparse. But we do not have to settle for so limited a concept anymore. Improved measurements of normal human structures and functions provide far more comprehensive information with far less personal invasion than in the past; we can define biological health as a positive state. The science and technology of the behavioral, social, and environmental sciences have advanced along with the physical sciences. And thanks to the wonders of electronics, we are ever improving our ability to assimilate large amounts of disparate information. It should be possible to reconstruct the elephant with considerable fidelity from its several characterized parts, even though different fields illuminate different parts of the picture. We must assemble a truly "whole-istic" view of human health, if today's Carelton Hensley is to have a shot at being like Hilda Echt.

So there is a primary need for an integrated concept of human health that is grounded in hard observed, measured, and assimilated facts and is contemptuous of disciplinary boundaries. But that's not enough. Health is best perceived as a dynamic human condition (or a spectrum of human conditions covering everything short of disease) rather than as an immutable fact. The WHO definition includes "a state of *complete* physical, mental and social well-being" (emphasis added).

Complete health anchors the health spectrum at the "north" end, but there is a lot of room south of that ideal before we get to a diagnosis, develop disease. Corey Keyes and his sociologist friends have espoused the idea that the health spectrum can be visualized as anchored at one end by a condition they call *flourishing* and at the other end by the opposite condition, *languishing*. There is at least intuitive sense to that. Even taking age and other factors into account, it's apparent that some people are happier and more productive than others, with no apparent physical reason for the difference. The adjacent figure depicts the relationship as a well-being spectrum between flourishing and languishing within the integrated health spectrum, anchored at its very best by the ideal proposed by the WHO. The figure deliberately shows a space between the spectrum of health and what we call *unhealth* (not disease per se, but the earliest deviation from the healthy state). At least for most of our lives, that transition can be avoided; it is not inevitable. In fact, given the chance, our bodies have an impressive arsenal of devices for keeping us on the good side of that space. Once one is unhealthy, the progression to disease is a very real possibility, but the usual medical approach may be able to reverse the arrow.

What is special about people like Hilda Echt, who "flourish" rather than just exist? How do the mind, spirit, and body interact, converging in special people in a way that confers not just health, but exemplary health? Is it possible to enable that special convergence in more of us?

No doubt physical health is an important factor. It must be difficult to flourish, hard to focus on much else, when constantly

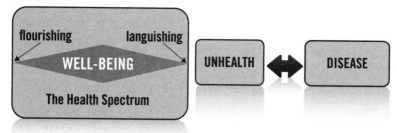

Ideal: Complete mental, physical, and social well-being

flourishing   languishing

WELL-BEING

The Health Spectrum

UNHEALTH   DISEASE

The Health Spectrum

haunted by severe chronic pain or other consequences of a seriously malfunctioning body or when subjected daily to the duress that a Baltimore steelworker in the 1960s would have felt. But what is it beyond the physical that sets these special people apart?

In *Flourishing: Positive Psychology and the Life Well-Lived*, a multi-authored book edited by Keyes and Haidt, there is a recurring theme that seems to transcend the physical (there is even a chapter titled "Flourishing under Fire"). Of the several words used to describe the pervading theme—optimism, meaning, fulfillment, creativity, productivity—the most inclusive is *engagement*. People who flourish have a deliberate and positive connection to other human beings whom they cherish—recall Ms. Echt in her retirement home dining room. This is not necessarily selfless behavior, and these flourishers are not martyrs. They "do well by doing good," get genuine pleasure from their bond with their fellow humans, enjoy the "benefits that accrue to the benefactor." And this is more than a state of mind. Remember, mind and body are integral parts of the same organismic whole. Behavior, environment, the things we can control are irrevocably connected to and interacting with our bodies. They all exist in the cloud of signals that fills the middle of that Venn diagram where we live. Flourishers are healthier than languishers.

Socially engaged people do live longer. Information relevant to this point comes from studies of men in Sweden. Engagement can be measured using several indexes of social interaction, including activities in and outside the home as well as "social" activities; that is, a broader engagement with people. Socially engaged Swedish men (it is likely that the conclusion is neither gender nor nationality specific) lived significantly longer than their less-engaged peers. That was true even when all other health-related information was taken into account. It was also true whether the men were born in 1913 or 1923 (and probably at any other time; those were the birth years of the two groups that were studied). There is something vital about mingling with our kind.

Complete health per the WHO definition is probably an unrealistic goal even if we could see the whole elephant. And as Ms. Echt personifies, the challenges can be in any of the diverse areas that integrate into the complete picture of health and well being. She had some physical issues, but even at a hundred her mind was bright, her concern about other people was intense, and she was probably no less rewarded by social interaction and no more inclined to hang it up than she was at sixty or maybe even thirty. Ms. Echt blessed the earth for over a century by her presence. She flourished. In the rest of this book we explore how a Mr. Hensley could also flourish.

PART II

A Vortex of Discovery

*With this profound new knowledge, humankind is
on the verge of gaining immense, new power to heal.
It will revolutionize the diagnosis, prevention and
treatment of most, if not all, human diseases.*

President Bill Clinton, June 26, 2000

CHAPTER 4

Health in the Age
of the Omics

FRANCIS COLLINS WAS director of the National Human Genome Research Institute at the National Institutes of Health during its phenomenal achievement from 1990 to 2003 of producing the first complete sequence of a human genome. He titled his two books on the subject *The Language of God* and *The Language of Life*. Whether or not you buy Dr. Collins's theology, his metaphors speak to the stunning beauty, elegance, and complexity of the genome's structure and function. That elegance and complexity continue to dazzle even the scientists involved in genetic research as increasingly sophisticated technology probes ever deeper into life's fundamental mysteries. Although the seminal accomplishment of drafting a map of the human genome didn't end the search for the fundamental basis of life as some anticipated when the effort began twenty-odd years ago, it gave new dimensions to the search.

Complete sequencing of the human genome transformed biology from analog to digital. Four genetic letters, strung into a molecular equivalent of words, sentences, and paragraphs, tell each individual's story, inscribe each human being's essence in every cell in every organ. You, uniquely you, can be identified from the sequence of those letters in a single hair, a couple of skin cells sloughed onto a doorknob, the saliva left on a licked envelope. Although you share most of your genome with your fellow humans (and to a large degree with other animals and even plants), part of it is unlike that of any other living thing. It is uniquely yours.

The genome project was completed faster than even the most optimistic scientists predicted, probably in part because of a race between public and private institutions (there is a well-publicized human drama there) to get it done first. The result was a maturing of the science of genomics. *Genomics* is the first and most proximal of an ever-expanding cascade of "omics" that is revolutionizing how biomedical discovery happens. We expand on the cascade later in this chapter, but let's start at the beginning.

Deoxyribonucleic acid (DNA) is an impressively long string of three billion units called *nucleotide bases*. The strings are twirled artistically into J. D. Watson and F. H. C. Crick's famous double helix (there is another human drama there; scientists, even brilliant ones, behave like real people) and then packed in a tight tangle into the nucleus of every cell (well, almost every cell; mature red blood cells don't have a nucleus). The strands are segregated into twenty-three pairs of chromosomes. There are four bases—adenine (A), thymine (T), guanine (G), and cytosine (C)—and the secret to DNA's power is the sequence in which the bases are arranged. A *gene* is a small segment of the long string of bases, and the precise sequence of the bases in that segment is a code for what a gene can do. What a gene does is instruct cells to make a protein specific to the code. Before the birth of genomics, biologists didn't appreciate the complexity of the process of generating proteins from genes, leading them to postulate that we had a hundred thousand or so genes, one for each protein. As the actual gene map developed, it became clear that the number was much lower, more like twenty thousand.

There are about twenty thousand genes in human cells. Twenty thousand different genes encoding different proteins. All made up of different combinations (i.e., sequences) of just the four bases, A,T,G, and C. The Human Genome Project figured out the sequence of the four bases in the entire complement of genes. The whole human organism is constructed from information made up of just four units, assembled in twenty thousand different sequences.

Proteins are also strings of units, called *amino acids*. Each amino acid is encoded in DNA by combinations of three DNA bases in a specific sequence. So a gene can be thought of as a string of three-letter words assembled from a four-letter alphabet, each word dictating to the cell to identify a specific amino acid. All those words (amino acids) are hooked together to make the final protein (a sentence, although without punctuation). More about proteins later, but it suffices here to note that their interactions and the processes that they influence construct the paragraphs, chapters and whatever more elaborate metaphor you wish (maybe a novel) that is the incredible, complex, and intricately orchestrated being we know as human. Indeed, a novel is a good metaphor: We each have our own personal human plot and narrative, each written in three-letter words using a four-letter alphabet. As complex as the final product is, the fundamentals of the language of life are astoundingly simple.

Announcing the imminent completion of the Human Genome Project, then-president Bill Clinton stood at the podium in the East Room of the White House on June 26, 2000, and intoned, "With this profound new knowledge, humankind is on the verge of gaining immense, new power to heal. It will revolutionize the diagnosis, prevention and treatment of most, if not all, human diseases." The usual politician's hyperbole is expected, but one is still impressed by the president's temerity.

A decade later, how are we doing? It depends on whom you ask. Let's start with scientists, likely to be the group most sympathetic to the situation. The journal *Nature* sought the opinions of a

thousand life scientists on the topic (the full results are at go.nature
.com/3Ayuwn). There was a consensus that the much ballyhooed
and anxiously anticipated revolution in diagnosis and treatment
of human disease promised by the president (and some reputable
scientists as well) has not happened. And these biologists don't
expect it to for decades to come (most guessed it would take a
decade or two, although some didn't expect it to happen in their
own lifetimes).

However, the success of the Human Genome Project profoundly influenced science. A large majority of scientists responding to the *Nature* poll (69 percent) said that they were either
attracted to science as a career or changed the direction of their
research as a result of the project. Interestingly, when asked how
the project had influenced the course of science, most scientists
said it was through the technologies that were developed rather
than specific discoveries. For example, more than 80 percent of re-
spondents thought the invention of machines and processes for
rapidly determining the sequence of bases in DNA, acquiring
enormous amounts of data, were major contributions. More than
60 percent considered a major part of the scientific value of the
genome project to be its exploitation of the computer-enabled science of computational biology, which spurred the development of
sophisticated methods for handling, storing, and interpreting data,
essential to extracting meaning from the vast amounts of information the project collected.

Was the Human Genome Project worth the almost $3 billion
that it cost? Again, it depends on whom you ask. Not surprisingly,
those most intimately involved in the project argue that it was a bar-
gain, the value of which continues to increase and will keep com-
pounding for as long as human curiosity persists. There are, even
now, some areas of medicine where genomics is used and useful.
Cancer is an example, especially breast cancer. Also, sensitivity to

some drugs can be predicted by genomic analysis; the blood thinner warfarin is a notable example (although it could be debated whether this has actually advanced medical practice).

But even its most zealous proponents admit the minimal effect of the human genome sequence on most medical care. "Although the effect of genomic discovery on the day-to-day practice of medicine has not been well quantified," wrote Francis Collins and his colleagues in a 2010 issue of the *New England Journal of Medicine*, "it probably remains small in primary care and non-academic settings." And none other than Harold Varmus, former director of the NIH and current director of the National Cancer Institute, was quoted in the *New York Times* as saying, "Genomics is a way to do science not medicine."

Varmus's skepticism notwithstanding, we still think it's clear that genomics has major potential for advancing understanding of human health and infirmity, but it seems equally clear that its clinical application is in its infancy. Some of the reasons for that lie in the incredible complexity of human biology. The genome has all of the basic information, but how that is translated into action, the structures and functions essential to life, is another matter. For that we need the next omes in the cascade: the transcriptome and the proteome.

The transfer of the genetic information from the nucleus, where it is cloistered, to the cellular machinery needed to make proteins, begins with a process called transcription (the language metaphors do proliferate). When signaled to do so, genes assemble copies of themselves, with the gene itself serving as a template. The genetic information is transcribed into a molecule called *messenger ribonucleic acid* (mRNA), which then exits the nuclear cloister to access the protein factory in the rest of the cell as illustrated in the figure below. Collectively, these genetic copies make up the *transcriptome*.

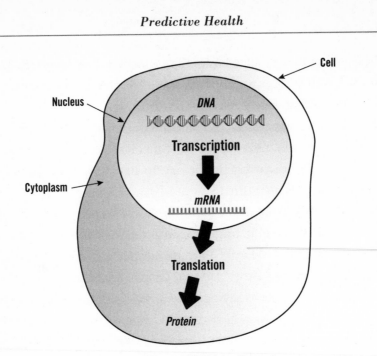

From Gene (DNA) to Protein

So this is sounding pretty simple, right? Well, it is except for a major complication. Recall that the human genome contains only about twenty thousand genes. However, the human body produces and contains many more proteins than that. A lot more. Several times as many. As is often true in biology, a deceptively simple fundamental mechanism is more deceptive than simple. There are several ways that a single gene can result in a vast array of proteins. mRNA itself can be modified by interactions with DNA and proteins creating more than one message from the original. And later events in the process of making proteins (discussed below) expand the possibilities even further.

Once the transcribed messages get to the protein assembly line, they are translated (yet another language metaphor) into proteins. Once assembled, proteins may be changed again by associating with sugar molecules, by how they fold up on themselves, and even by being split up into smaller proteins by other proteins. You get the picture. This is complicated. The collective population of proteins is called the *proteome*, and the science of measuring them is called *proteomics*. Proteins are the molecules of structure and function. They are either physically responsible for the body's integrity, or as enzymes, control the reactions of other molecules that carry out the vital life processes.

It should be clearer by now why knowing just the sequence of bases in the human genome doesn't predict everything related to health and disease. Genes are very important, but a lot of action is outside of and metabolically remote from their niche in the nuclear cloister. This will become even clearer as we move from proteome to *metabolome*, the hundreds of thousands—maybe even millions—of molecules generated as our metabolic pathways absorb and digest food, generate energy for cells, regenerate damaged tissue, respond to threatening invaders, and carry on the myriad other functions essential to life.

Metabolomics, the study of the metabolome, is an active area of current research. Although even the most sophisticated analytical technology is capable of detecting only a fraction of the metabolites that are generated, some patterns are beginning to emerge that have promise as tools for characterizing healthy processes and detecting (predicting) the earliest signs of trouble. For example, Douglas Kell at the University of Manchester, England, has used metabolomic data to construct a computer model that he claims can predict whether or not a pregnant woman will develop preeclampsia—the potentially life-threatening (for both mother and baby), late pregnancy complication of frighteningly high blood pressure—well before it happens.

Others emphasize the potential of this area for implementing the increasingly popular notion of personalized health care. The reasoning is that if each of us has a unique biology, then the health implications of what we eat, how we behave, what drugs we take, what we let ourselves get exposed to, and so forth are likely to differ. If we could measure the biological uniqueness of each person, at least things such as how we digest food, how we react to different chemicals, and how drugs affect us, then human health could be approached as a personal, custom-tailored matter rather than treating each of us as though we were a statistical amalgam of some large group (in any of those groups there is a broad spectrum of individual results that gets macerated beyond recognition in the statistical data grinder).

Although the idea of individualized (personalized) health care originated from the recognition that parts of each of our genomes are unique, it should be clear from the previous discussion that just having information about the private parts of your genome is not likely to predict the whole story. A lot of important things happen beyond the confines of the nuclear cloister. Metabolomics is attractive because this distal end of the "omic" cascade should be an integrator of the metabolically earlier events at the level of the genome, transcriptome, and proteome.

As an example, psychiatrists at Duke reported a distinctive pattern of metabolites in the blood of people with schizophrenia. Different antipsychotic drugs influenced the pattern in different ways in different people. It is tempting to believe that one could use that information to design a treatment for schizophrenia or perhaps other conditions that would be especially compatible with an individual's unique metabolic profile.

It is easy to be skeptical, suspicious of the hype. Scientists have become so enamored of the omic terminology that it is being applied to almost everything. There is now something called the *interactome*, which is supposed to include the complex universe of molecular interactions. Environmental scientists speak of an *exposome*, meant to include the health-related environmental hazards accumulated over a lifetime. Surely the nomenclature is a fad. But the science is not. An ome by any other name . . .

The challenge is assimilating the many layers of information into an integrated model that accounts not only for the pieces of information but for the networks that connect them. This approach, called systems biology, will make it possible to predict not just responses to a specific drug, but the course of an individual's health. At least that is our hope. We venture to predict that such new integrative models, built from the entire genomic-proteomic-metabolomic cascade, will enable us to predict personal health fortunes with a precision we can't now imagine.

At least some reasons for the contrasting health experiences of Hilda Echt and Carleton Hensley must have been hidden in the complexities of their respective omic cascades. Had those complexities been sorted out in the twentieth century, some pretty precise predictions could have been made. Things might have turned out a lot better for Mr. Hensley. Ms. Echt, too, might have been spared some pain and suffering.

CHAPTER 5

Taming the Wild Genome

THE WELL-FUNCTIONING centenarian Hilda Echt and the morbidly ill, sixtyish Carleton Hensley shared the many genes common to our species, but they also had their own complements of "private" genes inherited from their individual forebears. Some genes from both categories no doubt affected their health. They had some common tendencies and some unique ones, similarities and differences in their fundamental biology. How much did each set of genes contribute to the remarkably different courses of their lives and health? More important, was there anything they did or could have done that made or could have made a difference?

With the remotely possible exception of the few people who have a disease that is a result of a single altered gene, it is very unlikely that bioscience will ever manipulate the genomes of human beings in ways intended to keep them healthy. True, mouse genomes can be altered to discover how genes affect negative traits like obesity, but that won't happen in people, because most of the diseases that threaten us involve many genes and a lot of other factors. There are also serious ethical issues that transcend the technology. So, our genomes, like those of mice that are unperturbed by scientists, are destined to remain the "wild type." Those are the cards we are dealt.

No chance to discard. No new cards. Can't claim a misdeal. We are stuck with our wild type genetic hand of cards. But we can influence how those cards are played.

To explore the possibility of influencing what, when, and how much our genes are expressed, let's begin with the instant a potential father's sperm enters a potential mother's egg. That event puts an entire human genome, all the information needed to build a human being, in one cell. Somehow, as this one cell divides over and over, copying its genome for its logarithmically proliferating "daughter" cells (for some reason cells at this stage are always referred to as feminine), it doesn't produce a big glob of identical cells, but rather all of the thousands of different kinds of cells it takes to make a human.

The reason that one cell gives rise to thousands of very different ones has to do with the elaborate process by which expression of each individual gene is regulated. If genes are the words, the libretto of this biological opera, then gene regulation—to perhaps oversimplify the spectacular complexity of the precise timing, location, and sequence of expression of twenty thousand genes essential to the end product—is the score.

How does gene regulation work? Recall that the first step in the process of gene expression is transcription of DNA into mRNA. Transcription doesn't just go on willy-nilly; it is adjusted by proteins called transcription factors. These factors hook onto very specific sites on DNA, usually somewhere near the gene they regulate. Transcription factors can either repress or enhance transcription of the target gene. So the potential is there to allow development of many different kinds of cells and organs, depending on how, when, and where various genes are enhanced or repressed. You can see what a difficult job it is to orchestrate the action of these enhancers and repressors influencing twenty thousand genes in a logarithmically increasing number of cells, not just to produce different organs but to assemble them in proper order. That awesome task usually goes without a hitch and continues long after birth, as an infant grows into a child and then undergoes the incredible metamorphosis of adolescence into adulthood. It must require an exquisitely precise orchestration of a sizable fraction of the genome.

Genes are regulated, and if we knew how to influence that regulation, we might be able to play our hand of genetic cards, whatever they are, to our best advantage. Just because you have a particular bad gene doesn't necessarily mean that it will be expressed—maybe it can be repressed; likewise, maybe expression of good genes could be enhanced. The trick—recall the Venn diagram in chapter 3 describing where we live as in the confluence of environment, behavior, and biology—is to align the first two so that they favorably influence the third.

A veritable industry, based on a mash-up of myth, empiricism, anecdote, and some science, has developed around the concept of influencing gene expression by diet. Consider the relentless hawking of so-called nutraceuticals and myriad other foods and dietary supplements. Hoping to cash in on the sexiness of the term *genomics* conferred by the success of and publicity surrounding the Human Genome Project, marketers and entrepreneurs are having a field day. Google "genomics diet and health" and you'll get more than 651,000 responses (probably a lot more by the time this book is published). They include terms like "nutritional genomics," "diet genomics," and "nutrigenomics." There is even a European Nutrigenomics Organization and a company called NutriGenics, LLC. An endless list of supposedly health-enhancing products (often with stated or implied genomic effects) is available online (would you like a shot of Himalayan goji berry juice?) and in supermarkets and health food stores. Many of these products are neither rigorously tested nor seriously regulated by the government or anyone else. One query from Dr. Dennis Jones of Somalabs, Inc., to the Food and Drug

Administration in 2008 got this response: "[A] dietary supplement does not include a product represented for use as a conventional food. . . . The products identified above appear to be represented as conventional foods . . . and claims made for them are not subject to 21 U.S.C. 343(r)(6)." This is bureaucratese for "the FDA doesn't regulate these guys." You have to decide about them on your own.

It is beyond the scope of this book to critique this amorphous and expanding field, but we make the point that there is a lot of societal action around the topic. There is also some science. We focus here on some examples of the science and some observations on the practical potential of this area by the scientists involved.

An empirical connection between eating and health preceded any understanding of genomics by several millennia. There have always been foods that were thought to have specific positive effects on human health, and in recent times we have developed the notion of good food and junk food. But as we understand more about the fundamental role of genes in life processes, we can try to connect the effects of what we eat to how our genetic cards are played. Scientists call this *nutritional genomics*.

There are both general and specific implications of the diet-gene connection. One can construct a hypothesis: Diet affects health, genes affect health, therefore diet affects genes. Of course we already knew that diet affects health, but relating diet and health through the genetic mechanism adds something that really excites the nutrition people. They have good reason to argue that the "degree to which diet influences the balance between healthy and disease states may depend on an *individual's* [emphasis added] genetic makeup." From there it is a very short leap to the breathless conclusion that "dietary intervention based on knowledge of nutritional requirement, nutritional status and genotype (i.e. 'individualized nutrition') can be used to prevent, mitigate or cure chronic disease."

Attempts to connect specific foods to effects on specific genes are often thwarted by the highly complex nature of most foods (e.g., corn oil contains more than fifty specific nutrients, any one or any combination of which might be a critical genetic actor, if there are any). Individual variations in reactions to food further complicate any statistical evaluation of diet-gene links based on studies of large groups of people. But there are some interesting observations that at least confirm the idea that what you eat is somehow connected to what happens to some of your genes that are critically related to health.

Several studies have documented an association of what is often called a Mediterranean diet (largely plant based, little red meat) with lower risk for heart disease. But studies showing associations in large groups are always suspect. Whatever you choose as a cause of your favorite outcome could just be one of many things that differ among the people in the population being studied. For example, in the Nurses' Health Study, women who ate more choline (thought to be an especially healthy nutrient) also exercised more, ate more folic acid (another healthy nutrient), smoked less, and had a lower BMI. So, if women who eat more choline have healthier hearts (apparently they do), do we know why? It may or may not have to do with choline or anything else in their diet.

In the case of the Mediterranean diet, some more details are known. The diet results in lower risk of heart disease and lower amounts of several chemical markers of inflammation in blood (too much inflammation for too long is bad for your heart). Something about eating the complicated collection of nutrients in a largely plant-based diet results in down-regulating the expression of genes that contribute to inflammation.

Understanding the details of that phenomenon, and a lot of others, will redefine the term "health food," connecting the definition to the genetic and biochemical results of eating it. One can imagine a catalog of health foods that allow us to take optimal advantage of both our collective and our personal metabolic idiosyncrasies. Unfortunately we aren't quite there yet. The best we can do at present is follow more general advice, such as Michael Pollan's "eat less, mostly plants." But we are making rapid progress. Even if we cannot genomically personalize nutrition yet, the possibility seems real enough to be worth imagining.

Physical activity is another way that we can influence how our genetic cards are played. Exercise—or the lack of it—has profound effects on expression of a plethora of genes that drive healthy (or unhealthy) bodily processes. Those effects depend on what kind of exercise, for how long, and how often.

Roughly speaking, your more than 640 muscles make up over one-third of your body weight. That muscles are capable of dramatic changes in response to exercise or its lack is obvious from pure physiognomy—juxtapose a competitive athlete and a couch potato if you need proof. The processes of muscle loss (atrophy) or gain (hypertrophy) are a result of coordinated regulation of expression of batteries of genes. Many of those genes are involved in just changing the mass of muscle either up or down, but there are other, surprising genetic effects of exercise that are relevant to systemic health.

To be "physically fit" you have to rev up the genes that increase blood supply to muscle and increase how efficiently muscles can use oxygen to generate energy. You'll have to stick with a pretty vigorous exercise program for weeks to months to accomplish that. But there are some much quicker beneficial effects of exercise on tissues other than muscle. Even short periods of exercise have an antidiabetic effect, lowering blood sugar and insulin levels. In healthy young men, just thirty minutes on an exercise bike is enough to gin up expression of several hundred genes in circulating white blood cells. These genes influence inflammation (including inhibition of that response), growth and repair of tissue, and how we respond to stress. An experimental study found that exercising mice while feeding them a diet that makes them fat provokes increased expression of genes in the liver that help mitigate the bad effects of the diet. There is now even evidence that voluntary exercise changes expression of genes in the brain in a direction that would be expected to make the brain grow, improve learning and mental performance, and enhance resistance of the brain to physical insults. Apparently the "dumb jock" stereotype is not a biological phenomenon.

That diet and exercise have strong effects on how our body plays its genomic cards was not much of a surprise to those of us who spend our waking moments thinking about human biology. What did, and still does, surprise us (although it probably shouldn't) is that emotions also affect how genes behave. So what you eat, what you do, and what you feel all matter. The genetic opera is sometimes staged in the theater of the mind.

Laugh and your genes laugh with you. Laughter can change expression of a number of genes in white blood cells that are related to the immune system, growth, and cell-to-cell communication. It's not clear exactly what the biological consequences are, but the observation is interesting. We're tempted to guess that something good happens.

Negative emotions also matter. Your genes know when you're lonely. Researchers at UCLA and the University of Chicago found increased expression of 78 genes and decreased expression of 131 genes in lonely people compared to people who weren't lonely. The overexpressed genes were related to inflammation (remember that inflammation is bad for your heart and probably other organs as well), and the underexpressed ones suggested decreased resistance to infection. What seemed to matter was not how many people we know, but how many we feel close to over time. We're used to thinking of some definable signal carried by molecules to a cell's nucleus that provokes a response. What is the loneliness signal, and how does it get into the nucleus of your circulating white blood cells? You see why we're fascinated.

It is also fascinating to ponder whether the emotions-gene link works in both directions. Consider for a moment the love life of the vole. Only 3 percent of mammalian species are monogamous, and the prairie vole is one—one mate for life, come hell or high water. But the prairie vole's cousin, the montane vole, is into one-night stands and is very short on commitment. The explanation for the difference is in the handful of genes that the two species do not share (over 99 percent of their genomes are identical). The difference has to do with genes encoding brain receptors for two chemicals, oxytocin and vasopressin; prairie voles express those genes and montane voles don't. This gene expression-behavior connection appears to be a general phenomenon in monogamous mammals, possibly including ourselves.

As it turns out (you would guess that this is so), monogamy is not totally all or none; there is a spectrum, even in the noble prairie vole. And where one is on the monogamous versus not monogamous scale appears to be influenced by the degree of expression of those genes in the right places in the brain. It may even eventually be possible to determine where on the monogamy tendency scale one falls by doing a little genomic due diligence.

But this doesn't mean that monogamy or the lack of it is hard wired, even in voles. Blocking production of oxytocin and vasopressin in prairie voles makes them behave like their promiscuous montane cousins, and expressing those genes in a normally promiscuous vole makes it more loyal to a single mate. It's not difficult to imagine discovering nutrients or activities or pharmaceuticals that affect production of those hormones and how the brain reacts to them (we wonder if eating oysters works this way). But it is important to remember that the operative word here, as in all of genomics, is *ten-*

dency. A host of environmental influences have a major effect on sexual behavior no matter what hand of genetic cards you are dealt.

How your genome behaves is also influenced by where you live. The stuff in the air you breathe, the water you drink, the clothes you wear, the symphony or cacophony of sounds, sights, and other sensations around you—your personal environment—expose you to a world of modulators of your health genes.

Imagine yourself in two different settings where you hear a sudden loud noise. In one you are stranded alone at midnight in a crime-infested area of a large city. In the other you are sitting in the middle of the orchestra section of a lovely concert hall listening to Tchaikovsky's 1812 Overture, relishing the crescendo to the climactic booming of the cannon. Both of those experiences trigger expression of a battery of genes, but very different ones. Fear triggers expression of adrenaline, stress-related steroids, whatever it takes to prepare you for fight or flight. Elegant music (this has been called the Mozart effect) induces genes related to pleasure (and there is some evidence that it makes one smarter as well). Consequences of the two experiences for your biology are very different and in opposite directions.

Our genes are also affected by the less dramatic environments we live in every day. A Dutch study collected samples from 398 residents of various regions of Flanders. Expression of eight genes thought to be sensitive to some potentially cancer-causing chemicals (carcinogens) that were in the environment in different amounts in different regions was measured along with concentrations of the carcinogens in the same people's urine. Even after correcting for extraneous factors (like tobacco smoking), there were marked regional differences in the patterns of gene expression. Folks from Olen were very different than folks from Gent. And the patterns correlated with how much carcinogen was in the urine.

How those four genetic letters are strung together in your DNA—your genome—is pretty much fixed. Those are the cards you are dealt (or if you prefer the other metaphor, they are the libretto to your genetic opera). All of your cells have an identical genome, but those genetic words are sung to different parts of the regulatory score. Even the same cell will make different proteins depending on the circumstances—what you eat; what you do; where you live; what you breathe; what drugs you take; and even emotional stress, anxiety, grief, joy, love. Understanding how all the things that we can control integrate with biology and how to harness that potential—how to tame the wild genome—will give us the rationale for making health a truly personal matter. If you remember nothing else from this chapter, remember this: You are not a victim of your genome unless you choose to be.

How much of the very different health experiences of our centenarian, Ms. Echt, and the unfortunate Mr. Hensley, did they control, either deliberately or by accident? It's hard to say, but their lifestyles differed a lot more than their genomes. It is most likely that even had they shared identical genes, Mr. Hensley would not have lived to a hundred. Even a genome capable of supporting life for a century would not have been able to overcome the effects of where and how Mr. Hensley lived.

CHAPTER 6

The Epigenome

Disparate Identities and Kinky Mouse Tails

NATURE IS FASCINATING. Just when you think you've mastered some immutable rule, you invariably discover exceptions. Identical twins, for example, are an exception to the general rule that the sequence of the letters in each individual human genome is unique. Identical twins are really (genetically speaking) identical. They hold exactly the same hand of genetic cards. But of course they aren't really identical people. Their differences are due in part to how expression of genes is regulated. As discussed in the previous chapter, twins separated at birth and sent to live in different places, say Olen or Gent, would grow up differently, just as they would if reared in different homes with contrasting attitudes toward social community and exercise.

But separated twins would have even more differences because the process of gene regulation, the score to the biological opera of human development, is more complicated than just the interactions of genome and transcription factors. There is another level of regulation critical to human development that also helps to explain how two people with identical genomes can have disparate identities.

Stretched out, that long, elegant, stringy double helix molecule that is the human genome, DNA, would be—depending on whom you ask and how you choose to measure it—two or three meters long. That whole long molecule fits into the nucleus of a cell with a diameter on the order of millionths of a meter. Fitting the DNA molecule into that tiny space is not a random process. There is not just a random tangle of DNA packed into the nuclear cloister, a daisy chain of genes crammed in like passengers on a Tokyo subway. To squeeze into such close quarters, the DNA helix must be wound up into a ball, and precisely how it is wound up has major effects on how it functions.

DNA is wound around some small globules of proteins called histones, which—together with small molecules known as methyl groups, attached directly to the DNA—determine exactly how the DNA folds. This matters, because the way DNA folds can hide some genes so that they can't be transcribed: no transcription, no mRNA, ergo no protein. Changes in histones or in how many methyl groups are attached at specific places on the DNA affect how the molecule folds, making different sets of genes accessible or inaccessible to the transcription machinery. This possibility of determining what genes are available for transcription by how DNA is folded adds a sort of operatic *uber*-theme to the gene regulation story, another way to influence how the score is performed, how your hand of genetic cards is played out. The overall physical state of the DNA, with all its folds, methyl groups, and histones, is called the *epigenome,* and this mechanism of regulation is called *epigenetics*—meaning above or in addition to genetics—because it doesn't mess with the genome directly.

These epigenetic changes can be passed on to daughter cells and thus to offspring, including human offspring. That's very useful for building a complicated human being from a single cell. With gene expression correctly tuned—that is, with all the right genes switched on or off—to make a kidney cell (or heart or lung or whatever), this epigenetic mechanism can lock in the program, so that as the cells divide they stay true to their organ of origin and don't have to be programmed from scratch in each successive generation of a specific organ's cells.

Identical twins, siblings grown from a single fertilized egg that split into two with identical genomes, aren't really identical people in every detail, even at birth (e.g., their fingerprints are slightly different), and they can become quite dissimilar over time. Just how dissimilar is at the heart of the perennial question of nature versus nurture (although why it has to be either/or has never been clear—certainly calling twins identical betrays a bias toward the dominance of nature). What about who you are is hardwired at the start, and what is molded by life experience before and after entering your extrauterine world? Studying differences between identical twins sheds some light on that question.

Why don't identical twins, born almost simultaneously, die at the same time? Researchers in Denmark kept track of 2,872 pairs of twins born in that country from 1870 to the present. They found that how long the twins live is only moderately heritable; maybe 15 to 30 percent of their lifespan has anything to do with the genes they share. There are many other examples of disparate identities of twins (to belabor the oxymoron). Identical twin women may not be equally fertile and may reach menopause at different ages. Only one of an identical twin pair may develop schizophrenia or cancer. Hair patterns, birthmarks, moles, and teeth development can all differ. Height and weight and even facial features may differ and become more different with age. And identical twins may have very different personalities.

So the phenomenology says that identical twins are not identical people (the term *monozygotic twins*—hatched from the same egg—is more appropriate than *identical*, with its baggage of implied expectations). But there is a larger implication. If two people with identical genomes can be different, then the genome cannot be the complete and unabridged language of life.

A major reason why twins can be different people is that although their genomes are identical and remain that way, their epigenomes can become quite different. A team of scientists headed by Manuel Esteller at the Spanish National Cancer Center in Madrid studied this problem. They recruited forty pairs of twins ranging in age from toddlers to the elderly, from Spain, Denmark, and the United Kingdom. Questionnaires about their health, diet, physical activity, drug use, and other attributes were completed, and blood was drawn for checking out their epigenome. The twins' epigenomes were different, and the differences increased with age. The differences were also greater in twin pairs who had spent more time apart or who had different health and medical histories.

Whatever the ontology, the result is different people with identical genomes—disparate identities. It is possible that this apparent environment- and experience-dependent response of the epigenome may be a way for the genetic machinery to accommodate human experience quickly, adjusting things on the fly instead of waiting around several millennia for the sluggish genome to catch up. But it is also possible that not all of these epigenetic changes are just workarounds for dealing with the slow pace of evolution. It turns out that the nuclear cloister where your DNA resides is not as insulated from the outside world as earlier implied.

For example, a chemical component of a common plastic—something you may use every day—can alter your epigenome; miniscule amounts of it are enough to change the methyl groups on your DNA. The chemical bisphenol A was invented by a Russian chemist in the late nineteenth century. In the mid-twentieth century, chemists started adding it to polycarbonate plastic and some epoxy resins, creating materials so useful that over six billion pounds of the stuff are generated each year for making things like plastic water bottles. Bisphenol A—colorless, tasteless, and odorless—leaches from the bottles into the water and from there apparently distributes broadly into the environment. A 2005 study by the Centers for Disease Control and Prevention (CDC) found low levels of the chemical in 95 percent of a sample of Americans. The amounts were low, but within the range that experimental studies show can alter the behavior of over two hundred genes. We still don't know for sure what that means, but there are suggestions that it could have some relevance to everything from some cancer to obesity to diabetes.

Bisphenol-A isn't the only chemical that can do this. A lot of other chemicals that we are exposed to, either deliberately or by accident, can mess with our epigenomes even when present in miniscule quantities—arsenic, lead, nickel, chromium, some hydrocarbons, phosphates; the list is very long. There is much to be learned about any precise connection of these exposures with the epigenome and specific diseases, but the evidence is mounting. Better living through chemistry may well turn out to have many more unintended (and unexpected) consequences.

Even if you could avoid everything that might have a go at your epigenome, you still might not escape some consequences. The epigenome, like the genome, is inherited, so what your parents, and even their parents, and so on, were exposed to may bless or curse you with the genetic consequences of their better living though chemistry, regardless of where you live and what you eat, drink, or breathe. Likewise, your children and theirs may be party to the excesses of your behavior and environment. There is a scary moral to this story. It is not just greenhouse gases and global warming that threaten the health and well-being of our children and theirs, but also the very personal genetic legacy we leave them as a consequence of how we (individually, sure, but also as a society) choose to live and deal with our planet and its component parts. Ponder that for a while when you are feeling especially noble.

But the news is not all bad. As a starting place, consider the tail of a mouse. The tails of most mice are straight, but there is a special breed of mice whose tails are kinky. The kinky tail is caused by misbehavior of a specific gene (encoding a protein called *axin*) resulting from a misfolding of DNA. If a pregnant mouse is fed something (e.g., folic acid) that has a lot of methylating potential, her pups are born with nice straight tails, as though their axin genes are functioning perfectly normally (and they are). Assuming that mice prefer straight to kinky tails (that may well be a highly individual matter but for sake of argument indulge us), this story illustrates a good result of dietary manipulation of the epigenome. It is of more than passing interest that the offspring of human mothers who ingest inadequate amounts of folic acid are at increased risk for birth defects. Like the behavior of genes in kinky-tailed mice, the behavior of children's genes can be dramatically affected by what a pregnant mother eats.

The very fact that your epigenome can be affected by what you eat, breathe, drink, etc., raises the possibility that, much as the mice were "cured" of their kinky tails, something might be done to make people healthier or happier at a very fundamental level. In most cases, however, we don't yet understand in enough detail exactly what effects on the epigenome are likely to be positive; what chemicals, drugs, or foods might have those effects; and how to target the process to avoid doing harm.

To further illustrate the point, we move along the phylogenetic tree from mouse to rat. Rats raised by attentive mothers have lower levels of several hormones related to stress than rats raised by indifferent mothers. Something—grooming, licking, a pleasurable nursing experience—has different effects on systemic biology than does being ignored, or worse, mistreated. It turns out that the DNA of the rats with inattentive mothers is methylated differently than that of rats with happy childhoods. But, and here is the promising part, when the stressed and unhappy rats, mistreated by their mother rat, were injected with a chemical that reversed the DNA methylation problem, the levels of their stress hormones returned to normal, just like the rats from the better homes. These are rats, mind you, and we would not venture to extrapolate the specific observation to *Homo sapiens*. But the principle is an exciting one: epigenome-targeted pharmacology. Epigenetic therapies for some cancers have been developed and are in clinical trials. This is especially appealing because the drugs don't kill cells as current chemotherapies do—an effect that is difficult to target exclusively to cancer cells—but just change how their genes behave so that they no longer act like cancer.

We are who we are as a result of nature and nurture, not behaving as opponents vying for our persona, but rather engaged in an intimate and completely consensual dance, each leading at different times and under different circumstances. Influences of the two cannot be separated in any discrete way, further emphasizing that we live in an interactive fog of signals among biology, behavior, and environment. That is where who we are (and to some extent who our progeny are) is defined. It is also where we must focus our attention if the potential of Predictive Health is to be a realized.

The lesson here is that we need not be victims of our genomes. As we understand more about how genes are affected by behavior and environment, we will be able to more accurately predict the life course of a person's health and to design healthy lifestyles (or possibly new health-directed drugs) based on measurements of each person's fundamental biology.

In the meantime, we would give you very long odds that the respective epigenomes of our friends, Ms. Echt and Mr. Hensley, were much less alike than the sequence of letters in their DNA.

CHAPTER 7

Biomarkers and Biobanks

To BE A HUMAN being and live on Earth is to risk developing a disease at some point in your life. And there is an enormous list of possibilities; the catalog of human diseases used by medical people as a code (*The International Statistical Classification of Diseases and Related Health Problems*, 10th Revision) lists thousands. It would be nice to avoid them all and just drop dead (as our friend Ms. Echt suggested) of natural causes at a ripe old age. That may be unlikely for most of us. However, if we had some warning, a signal that we were at risk before things went wrong, then it might be possible to take evasive action and perhaps avoid the brunt of the threat. In fact, a whole industry is emerging that aims to do that—not just to characterize all of our metabolic signals, but to find the needles indicating risk in a haystack of physiological noise.

Collectively, these signals are called biomarkers, and only a drop or two of blood or a few cells swabbed from skin or cheek lining should be enough to find them. Not surprisingly in the age of data glut and proliferating omics, there is a spectrum of largely discipline- and technology-focused approaches, each with its cadre of enthusiasts. It's not yet clear which of the omics (or perhaps some other yet to be invented approach) will win out, but it is virtually certain that some combination of measurements made on biological samples and sophisticated electronic data interpretation will generate new models that will predict with reasonable precision a specific individual's health risks.

Given the complexity of human biology and the number of possible diseases, the magnitude of the problem is obvious. If you set about to identify predictors of risk for each of the thousands of known disease possibilities (plus an unknown number of diseases yet to be discovered), you have to assume that there will be biomarkers that are sensitive and specific for each disease. Discovering what those disease-specific markers are is the first problem (especially as they are probably present in very low amounts). The second is integrating that information with the other characteristics (environments, behaviors, etc.) of an individual person. The final challenge is the enormity of the task, screening not just for one problem, but for thousands of possibilities.

That might be doable. Lee Hood says that within a decade or so several thousand proteins with organ-specific origins will be readily measurable with enough sensitivity to predict impending dysfunctions. Our bias may be showing here, but you must admit that if there were a simpler concept that was less technologically demanding, the chances of success might be better.

Both teleology and observation suggest that theoretical possibility. The argument goes like this. Nature, at least in the realm of biology, is not generally a wastrel. Similar processes tend to support similar functions, even in different places. This proclivity of nature for parsimony suggests that basic functions of the kidney, heart, brain, and so on might share some fundamentals. If so, measurements of those fundamentals might be clues to health or the risk of losing it, in a general rather than a specific sense. And one would think that the more precisely one could measure normal functions, the better the odds of detecting anything abnormal at the earliest possible moment, long before blood sugar is increased, cardiograms are deranged, scans are abnormal, or kidneys start to fail.

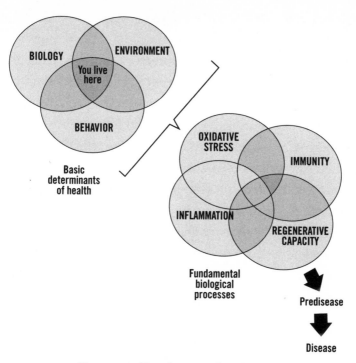

Processes Fundamental to Health

Measuring those normal functions is vital to creating a biomedicine that is about health rather than disease. If we could characterize these fundamentally normal processes and measure them, we could define (and hopefully maintain) health instead of concentrating exclusively on preventing each one of the daunting list of possible diseases.

Progress in that direction is already being made. Derangements of four interactive processes—inflammation, immunity, oxidative stress, and regenerative capacity—are associated with most common diseases (see the diagram above).

Inflammation is how the body coordinates its response to potentially harmful foreign invaders like bacteria and viruses. Once attacked, certain cells release a cascade of biologically active chemicals (such as cytokines and chemokines) that call in cells of the immune system to kill off the invaders. If it works right, the response is limited to the time and place of the threat—a precisely regulated assault on the intruder. But if the assault is global, not confined to a specific site, or the defense is insufficient to neutralize the intruder, inflammation persists. And inflammation is a potent weapon, intended to serve as a surgical strike, not a persistent holding action. When it persists, there are unintended consequences. Defense becomes offense. Persistent inflammation attacks the very organs that it is intended to defend. The eventual result is disease, the specific disease depending on which organ(s) are most vulnerable in a specific person and circumstances. Chronic inflammation is a prominent feature of atherosclerosis, diabetes, Alzheimer's disease, cancer—most of the common human diseases.

In addition to the surgical strike defense (that is, inflammation), the immune system has a broader responsibility for detecting threats to health and protecting against their potential to cause disease. Specialized cells of the immune system that circulate in the blood, with reservoirs in lymph nodes and elsewhere, recognize foreign invaders and generate specific antibodies that seek out and destroy the enemy. These cells can recognize an enormous array of potential enemies with striking specificity and react by revving up production of specific antibodies and mobilizing them. And these cells have the memory of an elephant on steroids; they almost never forget. Once it has been dealt with, if a foreign invader returns, even years later, immune cells draw on their phenomenal memory and generate antibodies even faster than usual (an anamnestic response; they forget to forget). This is why vaccination works. The vaccine has the right components of a disease-causing invader to signal the immune system without causing disease. That triggers an immune response that then protects against invasion by the real-world culprit.

As is the inflammatory response, this broader immune response is strictly regulated, aimed only at foreign invaders. But regulation can fail. For one thing, the system can lose the ability to distinguish between self and nonself and generate antibodies to one's own organs, resulting in autoimmune diseases such as rheumatoid arthritis. And there are more subtle breaches in the self/nonself barrier that probably play a role in more common human diseases.

We human beings are aerobes; that is, we must have oxygen to live. Myriad biochemical reactions essential to human metabolism involve oxygen. But as so often happens in biology, there is a paradox. These oxidation reactions, absolutely critical to normal function, also generate products, generally called reactive oxygen species, that can cause serious injury. When confined to the proper time and place, these molecules are not a problem. They even serve as the ammunition that inflammation and immunity use to kill off enemy intruders. However, when these species get outside their normal boundaries or are generated in excess, the result is oxidant stress, which damages normal cells, disrupting their functions. As with both inflammation and the immune response, perfectly normal, even essential, processes result in disease. And again, the specific disease depends on the circumstances and the victim's most vulnerable organ(s).

No matter how healthy your mechanisms for keeping your inflammation, immune functions, and oxidative processes behaving properly are, you still need a way to repair damage. Cells age and die and must be replaced. In fact, the cells that make up your body at age fifty are mostly not the ones that you started out with (someone estimated that the normal heart, for example, completely replaces all of its cells about every forty years or so). And cuts heal, bones regrow, organs recover both structure and function after all kinds of injuries. This involves a special population of cells—mostly residing in the bone marrow—that can enter the blood, go to wherever they're needed, and turn themselves into cells like those in the neighborhood. These are stem cells. We all have them, and it appears that the more of them we have in our blood, the healthier we are.

Of course the ultimate stem cell is that one cell created by a father's sperm entering a mother's egg. That cell has unlimited potential. The progeny of that one cell become an entire human. The stem cells that persist in adults are not quite that robust, but they can become many different kinds of cells. It is possible to identify these cells in blood using a panel of antibodies that can distinguish them from the many other kinds of blood cells (with the help of a very sophisticated machine called a fluorescence activated cell sorter, known by the scientists who use it as FACS for obvious reasons). Arshed Quyyumi and his colleagues have found that the number of these cells in the blood correlates with several markers of heart and blood vessel health, presumably because the more stem cells there are, the greater the capacity of your body to repair injury. We call this regenerative potential. There is still a lot to learn about exactly what controls this process and how it works, but much available evidence implicates compromise of this regenerative potential in diseases of the kidney, pancreas, and even the brain, in addition to the heart and blood vessels.

Although the association of derangements in each of these four physiological processes with common diseases—including atherosclerosis, some forms of cancer, diabetes, and Alzheimer's disease—does not prove cause and effect, the mechanistic implications of these associations are intriguing. There is also indirect evidence supporting a causal link between dysfunction of these general processes and disease. Behaviors that are at odds with human evolutionary history—obesity, sedentary lifestyle, poor dietary habits, and cigarette smoking—are all risk factors for cardiovascular disease, cancer, diabetes, neurodegenerative diseases, and probably other disorders.

Likewise, the fact that other behaviors, such as eating a Mediterranean diet, decrease risk for superficially unrelated conditions—such as atherosclerosis, cancer, and decreased brain function—lends support to the hypothesis that most disease is caused by similar dysfunctions of fundamental processes.

Biomarkers of inflammation, immunity, oxidant stress, and regenerative capacity might detect unhealth long before any organ starts to malfunction. The power of that concept is that it might not require measuring so many things that are difficult to measure, and it could provide a new definition of health maintenance and disease prevention aimed at fundamental biology instead of a specific disease.

Sidney Burwell, a legendary dean of Harvard Medical School, said that the hardest thing about teaching medicine is that one knows that half of what one teaches will be proven wrong in ten years, but doesn't know which half. The current pace of discovery confirms that statement but shortens the time frame. New and better biomarkers of health are always emerging. A possible way to deal with this is the biobank: "banks" of biological samples linked to all other available health information, vaulted away in elaborately secured facilities but still available for withdrawal and analysis for the future biomarker du jour, to the benefit of both bioscience and the biobank depositor, a return on the original investment. Some of the physical facilities are reminiscent of a mystery writer's description of a venerable Swiss bank: security codes; scrupulously secured vaults of thousands of bar-coded tubes of specimens in huge, refrigerated rooms with elaborate robotic retrieval systems; and extensive records of deeply vetted visitors, showing the times and locations of their visits.

As of this writing, the Web site SpecimenCentral.com (www.specimencentral.com/biobank-directory.aspx) lists 280 human specimen biobanks in the world. (For those inclined to nationalistic competition, the numbers by region are United States, 151; Europe, 77; Asia, 25; Canada, 13; Australia, 10; and Middle East, 4.) Their contents comprise a heterogeneous lot, including tissue specimens, stem cells, and blood specimens. Most are intended to preserve samples of DNA, today's preferred biomarker.

These are expensive undertakings. The biobank at the University of Manchester in the United Kingdom, which aims to collect DNA samples and health information on half a million volunteers, has an initial price tag of £62 million, and some have estimated that the overall bill may approach £10 billion.

One way of reckoning with the cost of building biobanks is to try to make money from them. Kari Stefansson and his colleagues developed a private company, deCode Genetics, with the goal of taking advantage of the unique situation in Iceland to build a DNA biobank linked to the extensive health records of that country's national health system. The ambitious goal was to include essentially all of Iceland's 270,000 or so inhabitants in the bank. An additional asset was the extensive genealogical records scrupulously kept by Icelanders. deCode made some interesting and controversial agreements with the Icelandic government and has built a large DNA repository that, with the other available information, has enabled substantial contributions to understanding the genetics of several human diseases. The business model has not been an unqualified success, but the deCode biobank remains a valuable scientific resource.

The folks at Vanderbilt Medical Center have taken yet another approach that holds some promise. They have arranged to collect DNA specimens from discarded blood samples on virtually every person who encounters their health care system. The specimens are banked and linked to the electronic medical record but de-identified. The goal is to provide specimens for genetics-based research, and the effort is supported by a significant grant from the National Institutes of Health.

It should be obvious that most biobanks as currently configured are research efforts. Most are aimed at discovering relationships between genome sequences and disease or disease risk. But biobanking is a young industry, still exploring its potential and suffering growing pains. The pains cover a range of concerns: technicalities of specimen collection and storage, privacy issues, ethics of information collection, storage and dissemination, data and specimen access, sustainable cost models, and ultimate benefit. There is a ways to go before it is clear whether the potential for benefiting human beings in their efforts to remain healthy will be realized, and if so, when.

The biobankers' infatuation with DNA to the exclusion of other potential biomarkers is also limiting. Although DNA analysis of large numbers of samples linked to clinical health information can associate genes with disease risk in populations, it should be clear from previous chapters that the sequence of letters in your DNA alone, except for a few single gene diseases, is not likely to provide the most sensitive and specific predictors of your personal health situation. There are too many other factors at play. Most current biobanks are not really designed to deal with those other factors. They are aimed at amassing large numbers of samples linked to clinical information to make statistical associations between gene sequences and diseases. The biobanks of the future should include samples suitable for every kind of analysis we can think of and even anticipate kinds of analyses yet to be developed. These would be biobanks with maximum potential to benefit individual depositors.

Altruism is a wonderful thing, of course, and if your biobank account can be used for the common good, that's great. But if interest accrues to the account, you'll want to be able to make a modest withdrawal. And that will require linking you to your account:

good luck accessing your deposit in the Great American (or wherever) Biobank.

Here's how the situation might look in a decade or two. When you first encounter the health-care system (maybe when you are born), samples are taken and deposited in your personal biobank account. You make additional deposits of samples taken at important points in your life (prior to childhood vaccinations, at the time of your first school physical examination, when you enter college, when you get your first job, etc.). High-quality standardized laboratories analyze your banked samples for any relevant biomarkers. All of your health-related records are kept in an electronic warehouse for your entire life. You and your health-care professionals have access to both those records and the banked samples as needed. To make this work—this is a real challenge—there are universal standards for collecting and storing the samples and universally compatible electronic record systems. All of the biobanks and record systems are networked for the entire country (eventually perhaps even the whole world). The electronic data system constantly scans the latest scientific and technical developments and relates them to your individual information. When there is a match—some new development promises to enhance the accuracy of predicting your personal health—you and your health professional are alerted. If you agree, the new biomarker is measured, the results are added to and integrated with all of the other information in your record and plugged into your personal predictive model, generating an updated health profile. Your health plan is updated accordingly, not because of an early diagnosis of disease, but because you can avert disease.

This of course raises the thorny problem of safeguarding your identity and its link to the intimate details of your health information from anyone you wish not to have it or who might use it to your detriment. Your account must be even more secure than your actual bank account, and you must control access to it by anyone who can connect you with the information that is stored there.

The topography of the health-care world can change. The rugged peaks and dark ravines, glaring disparities in quality and access to care, can disappear. The future Mr. Hensley and Ms. Echt can benefit equally from the science. Like Thomas Friedman's world, the health-care world can be flat. We are convinced of that possibility. But we aren't bold enough to say *will* instead of *can*.

CHAPTER 8

Zip Codes and Genetic Codes

IF OUR FUTURE Mr. Hensley wants to know how likely he is to contract some infectious disease—say Lyme disease—or whether he is headed toward obesity, it will be tempting to rely on sophisticated technology for the answer. Mr. Hensley could query his biobank account, have his banked samples analyzed for the latest set of biomarkers, and have the results plugged into his personal Predictive Health computer model. But for Lyme disease—and even for obesity—there is a simpler approach. He could look carefully at where he lives.

In some cases the geographic relationship to risk is obvious. If you live in northeast or northwest counties in California, for example, you are much more likely to contract Lyme disease than if you live in southern California (although there may be other risks to living in southern California). That's because the germ that causes Lyme disease is transmitted to humans by a particular species of tick—specifically the immature nymphs—and these ticks and their nymphs thrive in forests with special microclimates which are located in northeast and northwest counties of California. So, irrespective of the arrangement of the As, Cs, Gs, and Ts in your DNA, you're more likely to get Lyme disease if you live in areas where the ticks that give you the germ live and thrive.

In other cases the effects of geography are more subtle, but no less real. For example, the CDC determined how obesity and heart disease risk in more than 2,500 low income women was associated with zip codes. They characterized different areas using something they called a *use mix index*—the idea being that the more variety in the environment (high use mix index), the more health-related opportunities; likewise for areas where use of the land was very homogeneous (low mix use index), the fewer opportunities. Regardless of ethnicity, age, and educational level, not to mention genetic code, women who lived in an environment of variety were less likely to be obese and had lower heart disease risk. For example, women in a rural South Dakota town of 650 people with a low use mix index were twelve pounds heavier on average and had a 19 percent greater heart disease risk than women in a larger South Dakota town with a high mix use index.

These two examples illustrate the point that genetic information and other innate biomarkers will never provide all of the information relevant to health prediction; in fact, sometimes they may not be terribly important. Art Kellerman, former chair of the Department of Emergency Medicine at Emory, pithily observed that when predicting your health he would rather know your zip code than your genetic code. The phrasing may not have been original with Dr. Kellerman, but as that's where we first heard it, we'll avail ourselves of the alliterative opportunity and call it the Kellerman Conundrum. Even given that genetic codes do matter, there is some truth in the conundrum—people who study patterns of diseases regularly find compelling links between geography and health with compelling explanations including socioeconomic, nutritional, ethnic, cultural, and other environmental factors.

But, there are weaknesses in that argument. Zip code effects are statistics, derived from data collected from large numbers of people. Not everyone living in the high-risk counties in northern California comes down with Lyme disease, even if bitten by a nymphoid tick that carries the germ. And all of the women in the low mix use, small South Dakota town are not fat and at high risk for heart attacks. The same goes for the high mix use town; everybody who lives there is not thin and heart healthy. In both places there is a spectrum of weight and heart disease risk among individual people. It turns out that if you average everything, the theoretical average person in one zip code is statistically different from the theoretical average person in the other zip code. But it is quite likely that no single person in either place is exactly like the statistical average theoretical person.

You are no doubt getting the point. When people like Ms. Echt and Mr. Hensley show up for health care, what do the population statistics from their zip codes predict about their health? Regardless of where they live, they either have Lyme disease or they don't, are either thin or fat, heart healthy or at risk. Although fewer of their neighbors will be sick or unhealthy if they live in a low-risk zip code than if they lived in a high-risk one, the statistics of the group may not predict anything about a given individual. The big question is, how are population health and personal health related?

That question is at the heart of a very old philosophical debate among health professionals, sometimes articulated as the public health model versus the medical model. The public health faction argues for the most good for the most people. They favor imposing changes in environments and behaviors that will decrease the incidence of disease or increase life expectancy. Both of those measures, however, are statistical attributes of a population, not attributes of specific people.

There is a defensible argument that this approach—for example, providing clean water, flush toilets, good food, and lead-free paint—has done more good for more people than the individual-based medical model. A cherished example is the story of nineteenth-century anesthesiologist (and pioneer of the science of epidemiology) John Snow, who took the handle off London's Broad Street pump, stopping a devastating waterborne epidemic of cholera; by a single act he did more good for more people than the untiring efforts of all the doctors in the city. Eliminating factors that place large numbers of people at health risk has enormous potential to make society healthier.

Still, what about your genetic code? We have dealt at length with this question, trying to make a case against genetic determinism, arguing that you need not be a victim of your genome. However, in the context of the Kellerman Conundrum, a different question arises. Kellerman pitted zip codes against genetic codes, but how they relate to personal health may not be all that different.

A major criticism of zip code medicine is that it deals with statistically created people, not real ones. But the predicted health effects of genes are also based on population-based calculations. There are relatively few human diseases that are determined by the dysfunction of a single gene (like Huntingdon's disease, cystic fibrosis, or fragile X syndrome), and current genomic technology can confidently predict individual risk for them. But for most diseases, such as hypertension, cancer, diabetes, or heart disease, your risk is assigned by computer programs based on a statistical calculation, not your individual characteristics. The method is not that different from the public health model. In the zip code case there are statistical associations between some population health-related characteristic and environmental or behavioral factors. In the genetic code case there are statistical associations between a health-related characteristic and a population of DNA sequences. Based on that information, I calculate how likely it is that I will have the trait or risk or whatever relative to a large population of other people who have different or similar sequences of those four letters in the specific part of DNA being studied. This is probability, not fact. My condition is fact. Information from neither my zip code nor my genetic code as currently analyzed deals with me as a unique, individual human being in the context of my entire experience. Both approaches share the problem of the relevance of statistical information describing populations as a health predictor in an individual person.

Harvard psychologist and author Steven Pinker illustrates the problem. Although his genome scan showed him to have two copies of a gene associated with baldness—predicting an 80 percent likelihood that he would be bald—he has a full head of thick, wavy hair. No receding hairline; not even a hint of thinning on top. He happened to be in the other 20 percent. The statistical probability of his being bald based on the sequence of those four letters in his DNA was in his case useless, even misleading, information.

In a fascinating article, Dr. Pinker writes, "What should I make of the nonsensical news that I . . . have a 'twofold risk of baldness'? . . . Anyone who knows me can confirm that I'm not 80 percent bald, or even 80 percent likely to be bald; I'm 100 percent likely not to be bald. The most charitable interpretation of the number when applied to me is, 'If you knew nothing else about me, your subjective confidence that I am bald, on a scale of 0 to 10, should be 8.' But that is a statement about your mental state, not my physical one. . . . Some mathematicians say that *the probability of a single event is a meaningless concept*" (emphasis added).

We are reminded again of the blind men and the elephant. Are the partisans of zip codes and genetic codes both partly in the right and all in the wrong, prating about the elephant not one of them has seen?

The eminent (now deceased) Harvard evolutionary biologist Stephen Jay Gould addressed this issue in a typically articulate and insightful essay, "The Median Isn't the Message." After repeating Mark Twain's (or was it Disraeli's?) observation about the three increasingly evil means of deception being lies, damn lies, and statistics,

Gould related his personal encounter with abdominal mesothelioma, a cancer generally considered by medical people to be rapidly and pretty much uniformly fatal. After being saddled with the diagnosis, Dr. Gould discovered from the literature that abdominal mesothelioma was incurable and that the median survival from time of diagnosis was eight months. Told by his friend, the Nobel Prize winner in immunology Sir Peter Medawar, that the best defense against cancer was "a sanguine personality," Dr. Gould refused to resign himself to his apparent statistical fate. A median value, by definition, splits a population in two—half the population will do better and half will do worse—so Dr. Gould sought out his chances for being in the better half. He discovered that they were pretty good: he was young, they found the cancer early, he would get the best possible medical care, and he loved his life. He also discovered that the statistics were "right skewed"; that is, a few (a very few) people with this terrible cancer actually lived a very long time. The good news for Dr. Gould (and for the world to which he contributed so richly) is that he lived for twenty more years, thirty times the median. (Shortly after his original diagnosis, his death was announced at a meeting in Scotland, and a friend wrote a premature obituary, prompting Dr. Gould to repeat another of Mark Twain's most famous lines, "the reports of my death are greatly exaggerated.")

Dr. Gould's essay makes a critical point about the relationship between individual and statistical information. Our tendency in dealing with information is to look for "sharp essences and definite boundaries," which means we overestimate the importance of central values such as the median and ignore the "actual world of variations, shadings and continua." We tend to see the statistical calculation as the reality and the variation in the population from which the calculation was made as the abstraction. The truth, the hard reality, is the other way around. It is the statistical calculation that is the abstraction. Although no doubt a lot of people in that small South

Dakota town were fat and at risk for heart disease, it is also certain that a lot of them were neither, and it is quite likely that not one of them was exactly like the average abstraction. The hard reality is the information from each individual person who lives there.

Dr. Gould was not a statistical nihilist—quite the opposite. He found that his understanding of the statistics brought him a great deal of pleasure and encouragement that he would not have otherwise had. But a simplistic acceptance of the average (or median) predictions would have been abysmally depressing and, in his case, completely wrong. Statistical abstractions are useful descriptors of population data, but to interpret them without proper attention to individual variation is to risk making personalized predictions that are false.

A predictive health-care professional would like to know both the zip code and the genetic code for Hilda Echt and Carleton Hensley, but neither of those would be a reliable predictor of their personal health. Having both sets of information might help a little more, but predictions based on both codes would still be statistical calculations. Where the Echts and Hensleys fall in the spectrum of variability in their geographic and genomic populations is what is important for them.

Of course zip codes and genetic codes don't work independently—they interact, the one influencing the other. If we could understand the specifics of how genetics and environment interact, how each individual person responds to his or her surroundings, it might be possible to influence those interactions positively. Some of the remedies are general, good for everybody. But as we define individuality more precisely, it seems very likely that we will discover that two people in the same setting do not experience the same environment—the same input registers differently. In the final analysis, it is likely we will discover that your genetic code determines your zip code, and vice versa.

CHAPTER 9

Cyberhealth/Technohealth

Realities, Fantasies, and Myths

WHATEVER PREDICTIVE HEALTH becomes, one thing is for sure: It will be dense with data—data that must be collected, stored, maintained, updated, communicated, and secured. The magnitude of the job is enormous. Just storing, maintaining, and protecting data in accessible forms are challenging enough tasks, but even more overwhelming, at least to the human brain, is assimilating all those data, converting them into information, understanding. Someone estimated that the best of human brains can only handle about seven things at a time. Making accurate health predictions will require placing an individual's data in the context of entire populations, which means dealing with thousands of pieces of information simultaneously. In a report from the Blue Ridge Academic Health Group, Bill Stead illustrated the present and future problem in the following figure. The sheer magnitude of the problem will demand, as Stead points out, "new types of organizations, systems, understanding and technology." The good news is that electronic sophistication will not be the bottleneck.

Moore's Law, first proposed by Gordon Moore of Intel in 1965, predicts that the number of components in integrated circuits doubles roughly every two years; that prediction has held to the present time. Enabling far more than fun and games, digital electronic devices

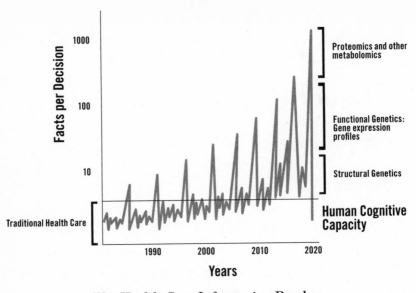

The Health-Care Information Burden

Source: Redrawn from Bill Stead, The Blue Ridge
Academic Health Group Report, October 12, 2008.

have proven potent drivers (and leaders) of social change. Likely not
even Dr. Moore envisioned in 1965 the world of Facebook, Twitter,
Podcast, Google, and Skype where we now live, although his law,
liberally interpreted, would have predicted it.

That may also be the bad news. We are immersed in an electronic miasma of all kinds of information, protected from inunda-
tion only by an available Internet connection, a tenuous barrier at
best (those connections are everywhere; they saturate the very air
we breathe). Like it or not, that is the world we're in. There are
positives, of course. Understanding and preserving health are being
revolutionized already, and we are only starting to imagine the possibilities. But there are also negatives. Alas, improved ethics and
morals are not implicit in improved technology. A fixation on hard-
ware and software can lead us to give short shrift to wetware—the
human dimension. But the fusion of high technology with health

care will create two domains equally important to Predictive Health: cyberhealth, which will dramatically increase the power of prediction, and technohealth, which will radically change how care is delivered.

As Bill Stead argued, we will need new systems to deal with cyberhealth. Already new ways to access health information have emerged. There are thousands of Web sites providing very authoritative-sounding information on any health-related topic you choose—from Addison's disease to the organ of Zuckerkandl. In 1999 a Louis Harris poll estimated that 70 million Americans got health information from the Internet; the number is undoubtedly much larger now.

And this is not just definitions, history, and other relatively bland (and not necessarily accurate) information from *Wikipedia*. Sites offer their readers the chance to evaluate the effects of drugs; match symptoms with diagnoses; get the latest scoop on a long list of diseases, common and rare; find nearby health-care resources; and even make appointments online. Who needs a doctor anymore?

No doubt each of us stands to benefit from knowing more about human health in general and our personal health in particular. That is true whether we are trying to find out how to do everything we can to stay healthy as long as possible or trying to understand the nature and course of a particular disease. And the Internet has made obtaining that information easier than ever before. But critically evaluating health information, no matter the source, is an important skill that takes some developing. Commercial Web sites, regardless of the topic, are often advertisers, sometimes veiled (thinly or not), and the content and presentation of their information may be influenced by that fact—those sites require careful scrutiny. There are other reasons to be cautious when conversing with these Internet health sites, including the possible mining of your information for other purposes—targeted marketing, information for insurers or for current or potential employers. The risk is often not very explicit.

Cyberhealth is also dramatically changing how health records are kept. In 1966, when our friend Carleton Hensley appeared at Johns Hopkins Hospital, his medical records would have been available to his doctors only if the care had happened at Hopkins and only if the records could be located. In those days, most hospitals kept medical records as racks and racks of paper charts, arranged by some arbitrary numbering system, and usually attended by a single clerk. Records could be checked out by any professional employee of the hospital for any reason—a clinical conference, a scheduled clinic visit, some special disease interest—resulting in paper charts scattered all over the place with no way to know where they all were. Often there was one clerk (out of the three or four needed to cover round-the-clock shifts) who had an uncanny knack for remembering the location of every chart, but that person invariably worked the day shift. The odds of finding Mr. Hensley's chart in the middle of the night would have been minimal at best. Knowing that, his doctors probably didn't bother to look for it, so a long list of relevant questions— Was this the first time his diabetes had raged out of control? What was his liver like before this? Was he allergic to anything? What medicines was he taking?—would have gone unanswered. Without the relevant medical records, Mr. Hensley's care, and most of acute medicine in 1966, was largely a seat-of-the-pants effort. This is a problem that computers ought to be able to fix. Presumably they will do that, but they haven't yet.

Cyberhealth is changing how records are kept, but the change is so slow that even in 1999, doctors in 99.5 percent of U.S. hospitals faced exactly the same challenges Mr. Hensley's doctors faced in 1966. Medical records were sequestered somewhere in a dusty rack of paper charts or, worse, lying unnoticed under a stack of unopened mail on some doctor's or nurse's or medical student's desk. Hospitals that did have electronic records tended to keep them in parochial formats, so that unless a person had always gone to the same hospital, his or her information may not have been accessible. Although the situation has improved since 1999, we are still some distance from electronic records as the universal practice.

Where there has been change has been in the U.S. Department of Veterans Affairs, Veterans Health Administration (VHA). The VHA has, in fact, implemented electronic record keeping so well that it received the "Innovations in American Government Award" from Harvard's Kennedy School of Government in 2006.

The VHA is the largest single medical system in the United States, with 4 million customers, 180,000 medical employees, 163 hospitals, 800 clinics, and 135 nursing homes. Back in the 1990s it started to design and implement a system of electronic records that made all data for each patient—lab tests, X-rays, examinations— available anywhere in the VHA universe. There are no medical records departments, no paper charts; everything is available when and where a patient shows up. Does that make any difference? Apparently so. For one thing, since initiating the VHA systemwide electronic record, the accuracy of pharmacy prescriptions is virtually perfect (said to be 99.997 percent, although we cannot vouch for the precision of the figure). Efficiency is up 6 percent as well. This electronic record system (dubbed VistA for Veterans Health Information Systems and Technology Architecture) is also available for free to any medical organization in the country that would like to use it.

As powerful as VistA is, it is only valuable to people being cared for in the VHA universe. The potential impact of any electronic record-keeping system won't be realized as long as the information is balkanized in different medical spaces. Common structures, with easy intersystem exchange of appropriately protected information among systems, are critical. As long as my health-related information is the hostage of a small segment of the providers of care, my options are limited, and my care is likely to be uneven, subject to the caprice of where I happen to be when the need arises. (It is interesting that even our government seems to have trouble taking optimal advantage of its accomplishments—Tri-Care, the active duty and retired military hospital electronic health record system, is just as powerful as VistA but doesn't connect with the VHA system. A current project aims to remedy that with a new, compatible system.)

These problems are soluble; the technology exists, it's just a matter of implementation. The bigger challenge is accurately and reliably converting information into understanding, synthesizing a body of facts that explains a system of complex interactions of an exorbitant number of variables in terms that help normal, finite human beings.

This is way beyond *Wikipedia* and the electronic personal health record. Major advances in health-related knowledge will coalesce in that ethereal universe, untethered to and so uninhibited by the limitations of fallible and limited human beings sequestered in their well-fortified ivory towers of academic or commercial expedience and personal ambition. One could fantasize that eventually the human roles in the process of biomedical discovery would be limited to inventing technology and gathering data—the computer alone needing to understand—making both the physician and the biomedical scientist obsolete.

There are both quantitative and qualitative challenges to such developments. Eric Schmidt, CEO of Google, estimated in 2010 that we now create as much information in two days as we did in all of history up to 2003. The figure he gave was five exabytes of data. We confess to a complete inability to grasp the magnitude of a single exabyte, much less multiples of them, but the point is that the body of data is enormous and the rate at which it increases is staggering.

That's true of life in general, but more specifically true of human health. In fact, one could plausibly argue that the rate of growth in health-related data is among the fastest of any area of human endeavor. Meeting the quantitative challenge will mean suiting up the cyberworld in a harness of health information and having all that integrative power make sense of it for us. It is quite likely that even health professionals won't understand how it all gets synthesized into something usable. The result can be a revolution in how health care is done that will rival the revolution in information exchange created by the device on which we type these words. The device dramatically expands what we can do, but how does it work? We haven't a clue.

The qualitative challenge is to figure out how each datum in those exabytes interrelates with all the others and to reduce the complexity, dumb it down, to human dimensions that we can grasp. That challenge is the purview of systems biologists. It is a qualitative problem because the way we assimilate information now and always have done is at best inadequate and at worst wrong.

Eberhard Voit, an eminent systems biologist at Georgia Institute of Technology (he wrote a book on the subject) puts the problem this way: If you measure a lot of things that are involved in the functioning of a biological system and try to infer how the system works by looking at each of the facts you have measured, your conclusions are likely to be wrong. That's because they aren't isolated facts, but nodes in a network. Say your doctor looks at a list of twenty or thirty things measured in your blood, and they are all "within normal limits." Your doctor concludes that you are doing fine. But you are not a collection of independent facts. You are a network, a system. Dr. Voit points out that every single value on your doctor's list of lab tests may be "within normal limits," but you might still be unhealthy. That's because each of those lab tests alone doesn't say much except in the context of the system that is you.

They interact in complicated ways, and if things happen to line up wrong, variations within what is considered normal in several things may still screw up the system. The consequences of small deviations even within the "normal range" may be exaggerated by small deviations in other important parts of the network.

What's more, not only is your biology a network, it exists within a larger network, the biosystem, a full understanding of which involves a higher-order network of different disciplines, usually practiced by people with different education and interests. Making sense of this can't happen in a human brain or even a collection of unaided human brains. It's just too complex. Engineers and technologists can invent and manufacture the machines that make the measurements. Data gatherers can stoke the cyber-metabrain with the bounties of their harvest. Systems biologists can suggest ways to go about interpreting the data in their complicated context. But the job will have to be done out there in the cyberspace cloud, beyond the limitations of our humble human brains.

Dealing with rapidly proliferating information generated by cyberhealth is only part of the opportunity for changing health care. Existing and imminent technologies can change the entire concept—what, where, how, and maybe even by whom health care is delivered. That potential has been called (not always sympathetically) technohealth. And, as in cyberhealth, technological sophistication won't be the bottleneck here, either.

The systems biologist Lee Hood calls this new era P4 medicine—for predictive, personalized, preemptive, and participatory—and various combinations of those terms have been used by many people to reflect the changed focus and the technologies necessary to make it practical. Hood describes technology that will measure 2,500 proteins in a drop of blood for modest cost, identifying markers specific for each of fifty organs. You can now buy a DNA sequencing machine for a mere $50,000, and soon for a lot less. The technology can put those measurements in your doctor's office (or maybe even in your local pharmacy or some other easily accessible place). What can be measured can change, and where the measurements are made can change as well.

Technology can also change the coordinates of personal health care, untethering them from specialized facilities and specialized professionals. A small start-up company, SoloHealth, in Johns Creek, Georgia, has designed a kiosk that consists of a seat with built-in scale, an automated blood pressure machine like the ones in your local pharmacy, and a computer. The computer records your weight and blood pressure, has you complete some health questionnaires, and tests your eyesight. The computer then summarizes your health risks, provides you with relevant information, and, if needed, refers you to doctors or other health professionals in your area for care; soon enough the computer will even give you a prescription for glasses and, if you want, order them for you. The records, stored on the Internet, will be accessible anywhere, as will the machines—grocery store, airport, wherever.

As in cyberhealth, where the computer promises (or perhaps threatens) to supplant the role of the human as scientist, technohealth is invading the territory of even the most physically skilled of practitioners, the surgeon. The robots that today remove your inflamed gallbladder or your cancerous prostate gland, guided by the hands of a trained surgeon, could take over the entire operation, banishing the surgeon to history's dustbin of medical curiosities.

Social networks, too, could take the place of the physician who is forever badgering us about smoking, diet, and exercise. True, smoking, obesity, and diabetes are personal issues—and the current infatuation with "personalized medicine" implies that focus on the individual is the highest good—but health is in a very real sense also a social issue. You ought to be concerned about me if I'm overweight, smoking, and diabetic, not only because you care about your fellow human beings, but also for the practical reason that I'm costing you money, running up costs that are shared by society at large. It is surely clear that individual people, even highly intelligent, rational people, don't always do the things they know they ought to do to stay healthy when left to their own devices. It is probably true that, as has been said of rearing children, making ourselves healthier takes a village. And there have never been in the history of our species opportunities to interact (network) with each other equal to those that exist now. The power of social networking can be harnessed to change the culture of health. Some rudimentary attempts are being made, but the yet-to-be-tapped potential is enormous.

Are we then headed for an Orwellian world of technohealth, delegating responsibility for our personal health and well-being to a virtual universe that connects to the world of flesh, bone, and blood only as a source of data, grist for the cybermill? The specter of robot scientists and robot surgeons might make it seem that way.

But when our centenarian Hilda Echt was asked how she managed to recover from cancer and, later, a stroke, she gave a lot of credit to her doctors and nurses. She said that their personal concern for her welfare, the support and encouragement that she felt from them, gave her the strength, determination, and confidence, as the folks in Lake Wobegon might say, to do what needed to be done. If we do it right, dealing with information (and transforming it into understanding) will be delegated to the cyber-techno world; the health professional, freed of that impossible task, will once again become the caretaker of an individual person's health and well-being. That's real personalized health care.

Although in this post-genomic age biology has been made digital, human beings are hopelessly analog. Information can influence how we behave, but there are other drivers. We are impulsive. We act irrationally. We are capable of analysis, but often don't behave that way. The technology will make this concept of a new biomedicine possible, but it will not make it happen. *Homo sapiens* will have to do that. We'll have to figure out how to avail ourselves of the best that cyberhealth and technohealth offer without abandoning our souls. We need more understanding of ourselves as individuals and as members of our species. Some of that understanding will be digital, a result of just crunching the numbers, but there will be no technofix for health. Passions of all sorts—love, hate, anger, happiness, ecstasy—are unalterably analog, and the picture of health is incomplete without them.

CHAPTER 10

Truth and Consequences

BIOMEDICINE IS RIDING an ever-steepening learning curve, but much of this new knowledge is not easily translated into practical use. There is no guarantee that new truths spun from this vortex of discovery will make us healthier. We don't even know that the consequences of new discoveries will be good—it's not difficult to imagine powerful scientific discoveries being diverted to nefarious ends. How do we go about discovering new truths relevant to health and making sure that the consequences of discovery are as good as they can be? In fact, how do we go about discovering new truths at all?

Let's start with the fundamental processes of discovery. One of the many quotable lines attributed to Yogi Berra is, "You can see a lot just by looking."

Some truths are obvious, there to be seen just by looking, if you know how and where to look. Ms. Echt's centenarian status could be readily documented. Mr. Hensley had a measurable disorder of sugar metabolism and its attendant complications, which we choose to call diabetes. Your blood pressure and waist size can be easily determined, as can many other indisputable facts. In many cases it just takes paying attention to the messages we get from our (aided and unaided) five senses. The art of physical diagnosis, mainstay of the physician for much of modern medical history, is based on a refined interpretation of those messages.

But scientific truth, including truth in the health-related sciences, can be elusive. The messages from our five senses, even when they are refined and listened to intently, may be insufficient or even misleading. Marcel Proust captured this idea in distinctly non-Yogian prose: "The real voyage of discovery consists not in seeking new landscapes but in having new eyes." The challenge is not only establishing the things we can see and understand, but also discovering new truths by seeing in different ways, expanding the relevant body of knowledge. Research ventures into the treacherous and seductive waters of Proust's voyage of discovery.

The generally accepted chart for the voyage, the scientific method, dates to Sir Francis Bacon's *Novum Organum,* published in 1620. Simply put, the process of discovery done this way consists of observation, followed by hypothesis, followed by experiment. Observation is recognizing and pondering the messages from the senses stimulated by the natural world and indulging curiosity, asking a question. Hypothesis is the articulation of a guess that might answer the question, a best guess based on what is already known. Experiment then tests whether the best guess is true or not.

Although this is elementary stuff to the dullest of students in 2012, in 1620 it was revolutionary. It was in fact so revolutionary that it dramatically changed the entire approach to discovery, a change that persists pretty much to the present time. Hypothesis-driven research remains a touchstone for most practitioners of science, and it has brought us to where we are in understanding and caring for the health of humans. Mr. Hensley's doctors knew that he had diabetes and how to treat it in 1966 because years earlier the Canadian scientists Frederick Banting and Charles Best had applied the Baconian method to discover insulin, which regulates blood sugar. The scientific method led Watson and Crick to the structure of DNA. There are many other examples. The extant medical canon was developed through application of the scientific method.

But advances in science and technology, especially technology, threaten the preeminence of the Baconian approach as the gold standard for distinguishing true from false. Once again, we can blame people like Francis Collins and his relentless interrogation of the language of life. The technology of genomics introduced an entirely new approach to science, creating discovery-based research in contrast to hypothesis-driven research. Sir Francis Bacon could never have anticipated it, but twenty-first-century technology makes it possible to discover truths that the discoverer could not have imagined as possibilities. No insightful interrogation of the five senses' messages from the natural world. No best guess. No guess, in fact, at all.

Given some early successes with diseases resulting from dysfunction of a single gene, biologists hoped to find the genetic basis of other diseases by guessing at what seemed the most likely genes and going after them—that is, the hypothesis-driven approach. But it turns out that genetics is too complicated for widespread success of that method. During an afternoon conversation in his office, Steve Warren, eminent geneticist, chair of the Emory University's department of human genetics, and discoverer of the genetic basis for one of the most common inherited forms of mental retardation in America (fragile X syndrome), put it something like this: There are twenty thousand odd genes, and any one or any group of them may be what you are looking for. For any specific disease (clinical phenotype), the relevant gene or genes (genotype) could be any one or any combination of an unknown number of unknown genes. In most cases no one is smart enough to guess what specific genetic aberration is most likely to be the cause of a specific disease.

Here's an example of the power of discovery-based research. There is an especially malignant form of heart disease called idiopathic pulmonary hypertension. For some reason, the blood vessels in the lungs get too small, making it difficult for the heart to pump blood through them, limiting the exchange of carbon dioxide and oxygen. After a while, the heart fails under the strain. The victims (typically young women) get short of breath and die before their time.

Sometimes idiopathic pulmonary hypertension occurs in several members of the same family. Some years ago Jim Loyd and John Newman at Vanderbilt University found some families in which several members had this disease and doggedly pursued the details of the family histories. They ran up huge long-distance phone bills tracing down every family member that they could find. They sorted through the voluminous Utah genealogical records. They made elegant color-coded charts of family trees and their interconnections. It was classic genetics—much like what the Austrian monk, Gregor Mendel, did when he compulsively enumerated his crops of smooth and crinkly peas—and it became clear that the disease was genetic. But they couldn't tell what gene was responsible until modern genomics caught up with them.

Drs. Loyd and Newman, with carefully chosen collaborators (Kirk Lane, John Phillips, and others), were able to show that the disease was a consequence of an aberration in the gene encoding a protein initially identified for its role in bone development. Who would have imagined that a glitch in such a gene would screw up the blood vessels in the lungs? This was discovery-based research at its most robust. Loyd, Newman, and their collaborators were careful observers. But they had no hypothesis that was relevant to the discovery except the vague notion that genes must be involved somehow because there was a distinctly heritable pattern to the disease. And they did no experiments, at least not in the Baconian sense. They availed themselves of incredibly powerful technologies to acquire data and then just went where the data led them until they figured out the answer. And the answer was something that they never would have suspected. In fact, the discovery forced a reconsideration of what the protein—bone morphogenic protein receptor—encoded by the gene actually does and how this terrible disease develops. In hindsight it may seem that the original discoverers of the protein should have thought more broadly about its potential function, but then remember Galileo—who had good reason to know something about novel truth—who is supposed to have said, "All truths are easy to understand once they are discovered; the point is to discover them."

No matter how new knowledge is discovered, there is the practical issue of whether it can benefit humans. It might seem logical to think that research focused from the outset directly at some specific human health issue—like diabetes or cancer—would be the most direct and expeditious route to human benefit. But that approach runs squarely into the same problem that bedevils hypothesis-driven research: the assumption that people doing research know enough to plot a course of discovery that leads directly to the desired destination, which is demonstrably false. Anyone involved in biomedical research will tell you that the trip toward new truths, no matter how carefully charted in advance, is invariably fraught with blind alleys, switchbacks, detours, and side trips, none of which was anticipated. Occasionally there are even unanticipated shortcuts.

Late in his illustrious career, Julius Comroe, founder and longtime director of the Cardiovascular Research Institute (CVRI) at the University of California San Francisco, and his collaborator Robert Dripps conducted a project that Comroe called his research on research. He surveyed the scientific community for a consensus list of the major advances in cardiovascular medicine over recent decades. He then identified the discoveries that made those breakthroughs possible and the motivations of the scientists who made the essential discoveries. Dr. Comroe detailed his findings in a remarkable book, *Exploring the Heart*, and in an equally remarkable series of articles published in the *American Review of Respiratory Diseases* called "The Retrospectoscope," presumably alluding to the old adage about hindsight being twenty-twenty.

One of Comroe's examples that everyone agreed was a major breakthrough was open heart surgery, the ability to temporarily relieve the heart of the task of pumping oxygenated blood to the rest of the body, open it up, fix whatever was wrong, and then hook everything back up in working order. The list of critical discoveries that made that possible is long: advances in surgical technique; advances in materials science and mechanical engineering that enabled development of the heart-lung machine; improved anesthetics; and not least, heparin.

When human blood is exposed to plastic and other surfaces like those needed to construct a heart-lung machine, it clots. The clots stop up the tubing in the machine, a serious problem if you're trying to build a functioning heart-lung machine. What's even worse, if your goal is to keep your patient alive, is that if those clots get into the body's circulation, they block the flow of blood to vital organs. That is fatal. No matter how sophisticated the engineering of such a machine, it was useless until the clotting problem was solved; heparin, which prevents blood clotting, turned out to be the solution.

The thing is, heparin wasn't discovered by anyone involved in investigating open-heart surgery. It was discovered accidentally in 1916 by Jay McClean, a second-year medical student at John Hopkins working in William Howell's laboratory, long before anyone thought of making such machines. In fact, it was not until twenty years after its discovery that any use for heparin in humans was discovered, and then it was to treat blood clots that form in leg veins after trauma. Medical history is full of examples of essential discoveries made by scientists who were plying the waters of discovery for very different reasons. And for every success of narrowly directed, goal-targeted investigations, there must be at least one failure.

The recognition that medical breakthroughs often result from research that is not goal-directed has important implications for how biomedical science is done. Generally, research is perceived as either basic or applied (and these days linked by the increasingly popular category of translational research). This structure implies a linear process, wherein basic discoveries are made by scientists who just want to know the truth, and other scientists who recognize some possible application for a basic discovery try to translate it into a practical context. Applied scientists only care about research that has a practical and clearly goal-directed outcome, so only after the translational guys have enough evidence to indicate that it might work do the applied guys test something new in the real world of caring for human beings.

That is a neat and useful way to think about discovery, but it doesn't always happen that way. Advances in biomedicine are rarely as linear as this model implies. Major advances in biomedicine often happen in a very different way that is less linear but probably more often successful. Such advances occur in a space that Donald Stokes called "Pasteur's quadrant," which he expanded upon in a book by that title.

Stokes recognized examples of pure basic or applied researchers, but he also saw a different way of doing things typified by the truly incredible career of Louis Pasteur. Pasteur was driven by both the desire to understand fundamental mechanisms and the desire for a practical outcome to his work. When confronted with the practical problem of an industrialist who made a living producing alcohol from beets, Pasteur proceeded to identify and characterize the fermenting bacteria and clarify the mechanism by which they did their work. The result was both a fundamental understanding of biological phenomena and marked improvements in the beet-to-alcohol industrial process (as well as the more broadly useful process that bears Pasteur's name). It was clear to Stokes that Pasteur wanted to

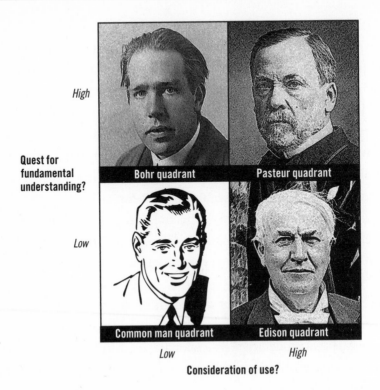

High

Low

**Quest for
fundamental
understanding?**

Bohr quadrant

Pasteur quadrant

Common man quadrant

Edison quadrant

Low

High

Consideration of use?

An Illustration of Pasteur's Quadrant Diagram

do it all, to understand basic microbiology but also to realize the
practical implications for phenomena as diverse as human disease
and the production of vinegar.

The above figure illustrates Stokes's quadrants: the common
man, not directly involved in developing either understanding or
utility in a scientific sense; the physicist Niels Bohr, an example of a
basic researcher primarily concerned with understanding natural
phenomena; the inventor Thomas Edison, exemplifying a focus
mainly on practical use; and Louis Pasteur, occupying his eponymous quarter of the diagram. One could argue that only Pasteur actually completed the voyage, discovering both natural phenomena
and their applications.

So the voyage from truth to consequences may be via a linear array of methods and scientists. Or the process of basic discovery and practical application may be intertwined in the minds and actions of a breed of scientists who live and work in Pasteur's quadrant.

This voyage will continue as long as human curiosity and creativity persist, and the resulting body of health-related information, already enormous, will continue to expand. What, then, of the consequences of discovery? On whose shoulders does the onus of responsible use of all this new information rest?

There are two parts to those questions: one is responsibility for the consequences of information revealed and put to use, the other for the consequences of failing to reveal and put to use information with the potential for good. The first is rooted in Hippocrates's dictum, *primum non nocere*, first do no harm. No sins of commission, please. But there are also sins of omission to worry about.

An obvious area in which consequences, intended or otherwise, can be negative is dealing with discoveries about individual people: personal truths and private information. As discoverers and keepers of those truths, health-care professionals bear responsibility for what happens to that information. There is an obligation to use personal information to benefit the person in every possible way, but there are consequences, potentially dire consequences, of revealing the truth. Can we ethically make those thousands of measurements describing a person's most intimate biology without knowing what we are looking for in advance? Once in hand, to whom does the information belong, its discoverer or its source? How can detailed information describing health in large groups of people be used to inform interpretation of measurements made in an individual without exposing vulnerabilities that could be exploited? What happens when something unexpected but potentially important is discovered? What do we do with information when we suspect, but aren't yet sure, what it means?

How research is funded complicates these questions. In the United States, the overwhelming majority of biomedical research is ultimately paid for with tax money. On one level that means that scientists are morally obligated to communicate the results of their research to the relevant scientific community. But more broadly, it means they must do their best to communicate the significance of their work to the larger body politic, politicians and citizens alike, in ways that resist the temptation to spin things to optimize personal advantage.

Then there is the obligation to enable health-related discoveries to be commercialized. We won't argue the morality of this requirement, but it is a legal requirement of people and institutions doing research on the federal government's dime. The route from truth to favorable consequences must wend its way through both the public sphere and the world of commerce.

Health-related discovery comes in many ways. The voyages from ignorance to truth and from truth to consequences are as many and varied as the people, knowledge, technologies, circumstances, and situations involved. There is good reason for optimism, given the possibilities that multiply by the minute, the virtual and real explosion of scientific knowledge and technological sophistication. Our storehouses of truths will continue to burst at their seams. The fly in the ointment of truth-enabled possibilities may be managing the consequences. There are expectations and risks to be managed, and care must be taken when reasoning from specific truths to general ones.

Realizing the goal of health- (as opposed to disease) focused and prediction- (as opposed to diagnosis) focused care awaits the discovery of the requisite truths and effecting their appropriate consequences. The processes that accomplish those ends are neither more nor less complex than any human intellectual endeavor. The promise is real, and the voyage is underway.

CHAPTER 11

Resonance

Research = Health Care =
Research = Health Care . . .

V OYAGES OF DISCOVERY are not confined to the ivory clois-
ters of sophisticated research laboratories. They are launched
in the clinic as well as the laboratory, in the very real world where
doctors wrestle with the myriad health difficulties of their fellow
humans. The enormous progress in biomedicine since Hilda Echt
was born and since Carleton Hensley lived and died resulted from
major advances in basic and applied science and technology, but
also from new insights into health and disease made by practicing
clinicians whose genius, passion, and curiosity launched other voyages of discovery. The best practitioners of the medical arts still ply
those waters.

Both the physicist Albert Einstein and the philosopher and
strategist Sun Tzu are quoted as saying, "In theory, theory and practice are the same; in practice they are not." That may be true for war
and physics, but there is an impressive history of discovery that argues otherwise for health and medicine. In our field, theory and
practice are so intimately connected that they, like conjoined twins
who share a head and a heart, cannot be separated without doing
great harm to both. So, at the risk of offending the memory of those

two great men, we would describe biomedical discovery, when the process is at its best, like this: In theory, theory and practice are different; in practice they are not.

Although various purely speculative theories about health and disease permeate history from the beginning of human consciousness, science-based theory in medicine has often followed the lead of practice. And practical experience is the only way for theory to gain respectability. One wouldn't want to be seen in polite biomedical society in the company of a theory unsupported by practice. Examples of how some major discoveries were made illustrate this point. They are also fascinating stories.

There was a theory, not all that long ago, that all human diseases were the result of an imbalance of four humors—black bile, yellow bile, phlegm, and blood. Now we spend tens of billions of dollars a year treating diseases caused by infections. How did we get from magic to the germ theory?

Although unrecognized at the time, the start of that journey can be traced to when a Dutch tradesman, Antony van Leeuwenhoek, first peered through his primitive microscope at what he called animalcules (later called bacteria). Leeuwenhoek had no interest in human disease; he was just fascinated with grinding lenses and building microscopes. He spent a lot of time looking at various specimens and describing what he found, "chiefly from a craving after knowledge," he said, "which I notice resides in me more than most other men." He worked in the Niels Bohr portion of the Pasteur's quadrant diagram (shown in the previous chapter), which may partly explain why it took two hundred years for his observations, reported to the Royal Society in 1683, to have a practical impact.

Then there was Ignatz Semmelweis. Semmelweis was apparently unaware of van Leeuwenhoek's discovery, but he was painfully aware of the death rate in the Vienna General Hospital's first obstetrical clinic. In 1847, more than a third of women delivering babies there died of childbed fever. What really bothered him, made him "so miserable that life seemed worthless," was something else he knew: less than 5 percent of women in the hospital's second obstetrical clinic met the same fate. Semmelweis was chief obstetrical resident in the first clinic. Rather than just brooding about the situation, he set about to understand and change it.

The prevailing wisdom among leading physicians at the time was that each case of childbed fever was unique, that there was no common cause. But Semmelweis, struck with the obvious geographical specificity of the disease in his hospital, didn't buy that. There had to be something shared by the many women dying in his clinic that they did not share with the women in the other one. The difference wasn't due to overcrowding; the second clinic was always more crowded than the first because Viennese women knew—even if their doctors didn't—that if they delivered in the first clinic, they were more likely to die. Semmelweis also excluded climate as a factor. But then he was stuck. The unexpected answer came with the death of a good friend.

Semmelweis's epiphany came quite literally by accident. His friend, Jakob Kolletschka, was accidentally stabbed with a scalpel while performing an autopsy. He came down with a fever and died, and the findings at his autopsy looked, for all the world, like he had died of childbed fever. Autopsies were the key: Doctors working in the first clinic performed them in addition to their obstetric duties, whereas midwives, who had no exposure to autopsies, ran the second clinic. Upon learning of his friend's autopsy results, Semmelweis immediately made the connection. Some contaminant was being transferred on the hands of physicians from corpses to living women. Semmelweis, unaware of Leeuwenhoek's animalcules, and without the benefit of germ theory, just called the unseen stuff cadaverous material. He found that a solution of chlorinated lime (essentially bleach) neutralized the putrid odor emanating from the cadavers and surmised that it would neutralize the proposed cadaverous material as well. Beginning in mid-May 1847, he insisted that all doctors wash their hands with this solution between performing autopsies and examining patients. The childbed fever death rate in the first clinic immediately dropped from 18.3 percent in April to near zero and stayed there; for two months during the ensuing year there was not a single death from the disease in Semmelweis's clinic. That was probably unique among the world's obstetrical hospitals at the time.

Despite this spectacular success, the world medical establishment did not accept Semmelweis's theory. They disregarded the practical evidence that supported it, and tens of thousands more women would die of childbed fever before a recalcitrant profession yielded to the evidence. Years passed. War came to Austria. Semmelweis, suspected of sympathizing with the partisans, lost his position at Vienna General Hospital. After a variety of other professional setbacks and the continuing failure of the profession to recognize the importance of his work, Semmelweis became increasingly frustrated. His behavior and mental health deteriorated. He died at the age of forty-seven in the Viennese insane asylum at Lazarettgasse on August 13, 1865. Only later was the significance of his life and work recognized.

Complete understanding of Dr. Semmelweis's discovery didn't happen for some time. Knowledge that the fever was caused by an infection of the uterus by a bacterium (*Streptococcus pyogenes*) had to await the advent of the field of microbiology, but he anticipated the germ theory of disease by several years. For Ignatz Semmelweis, childbed fever engaged both his head and his heart, organs shared by the conjoined twins, theory and practice.

Something similar must have driven George Huntington, a physician who, just a year out of Columbia Medical College in 1872, delivered a painfully exact and detailed paper to a meeting of the Mason Academy of Medicine in Middleport, Ohio. Huntington had been observing a strange condition in several generations of a family in East Hampton, Long Island. Beginning with uncontrollable spasms of the limbs (called chorea), the condition progressed to dementia and death.

George Huntington subsequently published his observations under the simple title, "On Chorea" in the *Medical and Surgical Reporter of Philadelphia*, the first of only two scientific publications during his career. We very much doubt the Middleport physicians were enthralled, but William Osler, the godfather of modern medicine in America, said of Huntington's work, "In the history of medicine, there are few instances in which a disease has been more accurately, more graphically or more briefly described."

But Huntington's description was more than accurate, graphic, and brief. Presumably unaware of Gregor Mendel's work—and certainly without the tools of modern genomics—Huntingdon described with astounding precision a pattern of familial disease that subsequent discovery gave a molecular explanation and a name, autosomal dominant inheritance. Huntington described what he saw with such precision that it paved the way for the later first description of a disease caused by an abnormality in a single gene. Careful observation by a practitioner, meticulously recorded, resonated over the ensuing years with emerging science and technology. Resonance: practice ↔ theory.

Those examples are distant history, but twenty-first century breakthrough discoveries confirm the pattern. Barry James Marshall was born the first of four siblings in Kalgoorie, Western Australia, in 1951. He graduated with a medical degree from the University of Western Australia in 1975 and began his tenure at Royal Perth Hospital in 1979. There he met Robin Warren, a pathologist at the hospital who studied gastritis (inflammation of the stomach), launching a breathtaking voyage that culminated with the discovery that the debilitating disease peptic ulcer is most often infectious, curable by taking antibiotics instead of being merely placated by major surgery.

From his own recounting of the story in his 2005 Nobel lecture, we can only describe Dr. Marshall's relationship with ulcers and the strange little bacterium that causes them as an obsession, perhaps magnificent given the consequences, but an obsession nonetheless. Like Semmelweis, Marshall's imagination was captured by the suffering of his patients, and he couldn't leave the problem alone.

Dr. Marshall was barely thirty years old and still completing his training as a gastroenterologist when he and Warren were first able to culture the bug. Once they grew the bug from stomach biopsies from patients with ulcers, Marshall connected the discovery with a long history of largely neglected publications that seemed to fit with his theory. Marshall was convinced. But there was a little matter of satisfying the larger medical community, who thought they already knew the cause of ulcers—stress, smoking, acidic foods—and the pharmaceutical industry, which had built a multi-billion-dollar business on the prevailing medical theory.

The proof of an infectious cause of disease has to satisfy Koch's postulates, four rules established by Robert Koch and Friedrich Loeffler in the late nineteenth century. Marshall and Warren's work met all of the rules except one: that administration of a pure culture of the offending agent must cause the disease when given to a susceptible host. So Dr. Marshall had his colleague make a slurry of a pure culture of a *Helicobacter pylori*, and Marshall drank it. (In a cartoon panel that is part of Marshall's Nobel lecture, his assistant yells, "You're crazy," to which Marshall replies, brandishing the beaker of green slurry, "There's no other way." Marshall commented, "In 1984, both statements were true enough.") Marshall had no symptoms for several days, and he pondered whether the self-experiment had failed, whether he was destined to spend the rest of his life in the private practice of gastroenterology in some obscure Australian outpost, a scientific pariah. But after a week or so he developed the symptoms of gastritis, confirmed by a biopsy. Koch's criteria for proof of cause were satisfied.

Most ulcers are now cured with antibiotics. The diagnosis is no longer a life sentence that raises the specter of sudden fatal hemorrhage or major surgical manipulations of significant portions of the gastrointestinal tract. *H. pylori* was indeed Dr. Marshall's magnificent obsession.

In this country, career tracks for physicians have become separated into either practicing doctor or what is usually referred to as physician scientist. It's either/or. And, at least if we take grant-funding statistics as a measure of success, the physician scientist is a vanishing breed. During the years 1996–2003, a boom time for the National Institutes of Health, the number of PhDs applying for grants for the first time increased 43 percent, while the number of MDs decreased 4 percent. The picture is even bleaker now. Real advances in biomedicine need physician scientists to bring both the perspective of practice and scientific rigor to the task. The most fecund sources of discovery are teams of scientists and practitioners.

We caution against too rigid a structure and too narrow expectations of the MD. This child of discovery may not thrive by being so strictly divided. King Solomon would have seen it: the child of discovery cannot be severed in two without serious injury. Resonance and dissonance are different creatures. One task of Predictive Health is to dull the too bright line that has been drawn between the laboratory and the clinic.

It is not news that human health is a complicated business—so complicated that decisions about health are almost always made with incomplete information. If we pay attention, we learn from the consequences of those decisions, good or bad, so that we capture our successes and don't repeat our mistakes. That is acquiring new knowledge, and acquiring new knowledge is research. At least in the modern world of biomedicine, health care is research. When it works best, information from clinical experience and new information from the laboratory inform each other, enriching the process, making it more productive and more efficient. The essential resonance between the laboratory and the clinic is why physicians must be committed to and intimately engaged in the process of discovery. The linear model of basic research to translational research to clinical trials fails us.

The failure should be obvious. Basic discoveries may have immediate implications for health care—one could even argue that, morally, they should be applied, and as quickly as possible. Also, as with Semmelweis and Huntington, all kinds of information must flow from patients to inform questions that basic science addresses. A vigorous conversation between basic and clinical scientists (which all doctors are if they are doing their jobs) is essential to discovery and to the subsequent refinement of new knowledge into practicable form.

There is much yet to be discovered about human health if the paradigm is to shift from curing disease to keeping ourselves healthy. Those discoveries will not happen in ivory academic towers isolated from the complex world where biology, behavior, and environment meld. Those of us taking on the task of caring for health must, like Ignatz Semmelweis, engage our keenest senses and our deepest concerns about our fellows, observe and communicate what we encounter as meticulously as George Huntington did, and defy conventional wisdom with the obsessive tenacity of a Barry Marshall if we are to realize the possibilities.

In theory, theory and practice are different; in practice they are not.

PART III

Health vis-à-vis Disease

Moving the Target

*So much for the theory and the tools—
existing or soon to come—that will make
Predictive Health possible. But what would it
look like in practice in the real world?*

CHAPTER 12

The Devils We Know

CARLETON HENSLEY'S diabetes and high blood pressure should have been treated earlier and more aggressively; had that been done, he would have lived a better life, longer than he did. But in the Predictive Health world, we wouldn't wait for him to get a disease, that would be missing the big opportunity to prevent it. It may seem from previous chapters that we don't yet have all the tools to completely predict Mr. Hensley's health, and that is true, but even now there are some opportunities for focusing on and keeping health that don't require new science and new machines.

Some things that predict health and the risk of losing it are pretty easy to measure. Waist size is a good example. We are fat and getting fatter, literally feeding an epidemic of type II diabetes the likes of which the world has never seen. The story is even bleaker than that: Obesity leads to diabetes, but also results in too much fat in the blood, high blood pressure, and heart disease. There is even a name for it—metabolic syndrome. The story of how we got here is complex, but there are some explanations.

In midafternoon on a crisp December day in 2005, the author Tom Wolfe sat with a panel of biomedical scientists at the first annual Emory Georgia Tech Predictive Health Symposium. He was asked, "Mr. Wolfe, how do you define health?"

"I rely a lot on denial," he answered.

An amusing answer, but perhaps—if Tom Wolfe shares the foibles of his fellow humans about whom he writes (one suspects that he does)—a more candid one than the audience appreciated. When it comes to health, denial must be a common attitude. How else do we explain why, among other things, we (both the personal we and the social we) are misbehaving ourselves into an epidemic of obesity and its myriad complications. Disconnecting behavior from consequences is a convenient device for marketing overindulgence, but it doesn't change the facts. We must be denying them.

There are some statistical facts that define the problem and describe its chronology. Close to a third of Americans are obese. Obesity is not just carrying a few pounds more than our ideal weight (although another third of Americans fit that description). Obesity is officially defined as having a body mass index (BMI, i.e., weight adjusted for height) greater than 30. For a person of average height, that translates roughly into more than thirty excess pounds, and a consequent increased risk of diabetes, heart attack, high blood pressure, physical injury, cancer, and probably Alzheimer's disease. The list continues to grow.

The epidemic started only recently and is rapidly expanding. Between 1980 and 2000 the prevalence of obese Americans doubled (from 15 to 30 percent of the population); the fraction that was either overweight or obese increased from half to two-thirds. And the expansion of the problem continues apace. This is an expensive proposition. Health policy expert Ken Thorpe calculates that more than a quarter of the increase in health-care costs in the United States over the past several years is a direct result of obesity and its associated ills. We all share those costs. This epidemic is a concern for all of us whether or not we are personally participating in it.

There are also both biological and cultural facts that bear on the problem. For one thing, there is the "omnivore's dilemma," as Michael Pollan described the difficulty deciding what's for dinner for a species that can eat anything. The Emory anthropologist George Armelagos argues that our species' biocultural answer to the problem is the genesis of the epidemic.

Armelagos opens his argument, published in *Journal of Anthropological Research*, with a quote from *Winnie-the-Pooh*. Piglet asks his friend Pooh what he first says to himself when he wakes up in the morning. Pooh answers, "What's for breakfast?" Piglet responds that he says, "I wonder what's going to happen exciting today?" After a moment's thought, Pooh concludes that the two answers mean the same thing.

The concerns of our Neolithic forebears (and our concerns) are necessarily more akin to those of Pooh than Piglet. We can live and reproduce (although perhaps not flourish) without exciting experiences. But we must eat, and in sufficient quality and quantity. Our omnivore's advantage is that we can eat anything, but the dilemma is getting the right amount of the good stuff while avoiding the bad stuff.

The "bio" part of the biocultural solution with which we are saddled, Armelagos argues, includes the evolution of large brains and small digestive tracts. Large brains are nutritionally expensive (our brain accounts for 2 percent of our body but 20 percent of our energy use). Small digestive tracts mean that we need nutritionally denser and more readily digestible foods. Our cultural response was to develop a cuisine that decreased diversity and emphasized preparation, taste, and so on, making eating an esthetic experience and disconnecting eating behavior from the biological imperative. From there it was a straight shot to mass production and marketing of cheap, calorie- and fat-dense foods, available with little effort, an easy sell to two-job families with mouths to feed and pressed for time.

Then there is Greg Gibson's genetic argument (akin to but distinct from the thrifty gene hypothesis, which blames our outdated metabolic tendency to store up fat in anticipation of hard times, necessary in a resource-poor, primitive milieu but unnecessary in our world of plenty). In *It Takes a Genome,* Gibson opines that we have simply outpaced our genes. Our genome lumbers along its evolutionary course at a millennial pace, while in just a few short decades we have freed ourselves of the need for physical exertion and pampered our short digestive tracts with excesses of readily available calories, fats, and the like. The result: Our genome is "out of equilibrium with itself and with the environment," in Gibson's words. The marvelous, genetically dictated metabolic apparatus that worked fine throughout most of primate history is a bad fit for how we have chosen to live now. The mismatch makes us suddenly (at least in evolutionary terms) vulnerable to the catalog of failing organs listed previously. We may be able to blame our sluggishly evolving genome for the epidemic, at least as a species, but that doesn't work so well for individuals.

Maybe the biocultural solution to the omnivore's dilemma and a sluggishly adjusting genome help explain why there is an epidemic, but they don't explain why only some of us are fat and unhealthy. Individual differences in our biology might be part of the explanation.

No doubt Hilda Echt, lean and reasonably active at a hundred, and Carleton Hensley, overweight with high blood pressure and diabetes at little more than half that age, had some differences in their basic biology. And no doubt some of those differences were in their DNA. Although Ms. Echt's and Mr. Hensley's genomes were 99.6 percent identical, as are all of our genomes, it is certain that Ms. Echt's and Mr. Hensley's very different ancestors contributed some different genes to each of them. There could be some comfort in believing that one's BMI is coded in an immutable genome, that fat and skinny are destinies; to be able to bless (or damn) parents, grandparents, and more remote members of the family tree for one's physiognomy.

Geneticists have made some progress in this area. For example, obesity in a few (vanishingly few) people is the result of a specific identifiable genetic abnormality. Some people have a glitch in a gene encoding a hormone called leptin, which is made by normal fat cells and signals the brain to stop eating. People who can't make leptin have ravenous appetites and become obese, but the problem can be treated successfully with injections of the hormone. Some other genes do seem to be involved in regulating body fat, but we don't yet have the information that makes straightforward connections between their structure and function and an individual's BMI.

The *New York Times* science writer Gina Kolata, in *Rethinking Thin*, cites the familial tendency to obesity, the frequent failure of diets (at least in the long run), and recent genetic discoveries to make her case that genetic predestination may be a major explanation for the problem. Maybe it's not an epidemic at all, but a medico-media overreaction to an inevitably changing physiognomy with minimal health implications. Although there is no doubt that some people are more prone to be obese than others and that it is likely some of that proclivity is in their DNA, the larger argument is difficult to swallow.

For one thing, the epidemic is only a few decades old, so, given the pace of evolution, the doubling of obesity rates in the United States over twenty years cannot possibly be a result of changes in our collective genome. Also, minimizing the relationship between obesity and serious disease ignores the unassailable facts. Although being overweight or obese is not a moral issue, and some of us are more susceptible than others, the fact remains that this epidemic is the most serious health challenge in this country, and it continues to worsen.

Clearly the biology is important, but recall that environment and behavior interact with biology to make us who we are. And our environment a) encourages inactivity—there are towns with few sidewalks, shops are too far from home to walk there anyway, and computer games have replaced hide-and-seek or kick-the-can; b) makes unhealthy food cheap and available (requiring so little preparation that it scarcely distracts us from the ubiquitous computer or is even handed to us at a drive-through window, barely disturbing us in the comfort of our car); and c) aggressively markets that lifestyle.

There may also be some more fundamental determinants of how we behave. At the Yerkes Primate Center's bucolic retreat outside of Atlanta, a colony of monkeys live and breed much as they would do in the wild. These primates are unexposed to and uninfluenced by Madison Avenue hype and Hollywood stereotypes. They don't watch TV; they don't read *People* magazine (or any monkey equivalent). There is no nonhuman primate cinema. The fashion runways of Milan and New York with their skeletal models are completely foreign to these guys. They are oblivious to the barrage of medico-media handwringing about obesity and its complications. They are just monkeys behaving like monkeys.

It turns out that monkeys behaving like monkeys develop an interesting and complex social order. There are dominant groups and submissive groups, and they eat differently. Given the same unlimited access to regular monkey chow, the dominant animals eat more than the submissive ones, but they don't overeat. The monkeys are not obese. However, when all of the animals are provided with unlimited access to the monkey equivalent of comfort food (some kind of banana-flavored, calorie-dense fare that tastes pretty good even to a human) in addition to the healthy monkey chow, the submissive group eats a lot more of the comfort food than the dominant group does. A lot more. The submissive monkeys stay up at night eating this stuff. And they get fat.

The explanation is stress. Being a submissive monkey is stressful. And stress affects what and how much they eat, even absent the myriad other environmental influences that we humans must deal with. And here's the scariest part of the story. Take away the comfort food, and the submissive monkeys keep overeating even the ordinary monkey food. That rich stuff does something to the brain that transcends the immediate effects of the high-calorie food.

A great monkey story, right? But we aren't monkeys (although some of our behaviors might challenge that assertion). What if we do a similar experiment with people? Seat a group of ordinary people around a table in a room with bowls of M&Ms and similar bowls of red grapes on the table. Give each of them an anagram to solve. Unknown to the participants in this little ruse, by random assignment, half of the people get an easily solvable anagram and half get an impossible one. The group with the easy anagrams go for the grapes, and the ones with the impossible task go for the M&Ms. Stress, even short-term, trivial stress, affects what and how much we choose to eat. And that's not even taking into account availability, cost, and all the other relevant variables. Expand those observations into the larger human experience and ponder the implications of the lasting effects on eating behavior that we saw in the monkeys, and it's not very difficult to imagine that we have the makings of an epidemic.

All of this is very interesting, even alarming, but maybe you are thinking that your BMI is in the middle of the normal range; you're not part of the problem. Your socially conscious side is concerned, but you don't personally have to worry about it. Sorry to break the news, but to borrow a line from *Porgy and Bess*, it ain't necessarily so.

What seems to be emerging from several epidemiological studies (from Mayo, Harvard, and elsewhere) is that fat, not body weight or BMI, is the culprit. And here's the unexpected news: it's not the absolute amount of fat, but the amount relative to the total size of one's body. This is often reflected in total body weight (or BMI) for people who are overweight, because when most people gain weight, they gain mostly fat. But it is possible to have a normal body weight and still be too fat in relative terms, which turns out to be a fairly common problem.

In a study underway at the Emory Georgia Tech Center for Health Discovery and Well Being®, approximately seven hundred individuals—randomly chosen, working full time, and essentially healthy—are being evaluated in detail: mentally, socially, physically, and spiritually. Among other measures, their body composition (especially percent body fat) is measured by a low radiation whole-body scan. About two-thirds of these people are overweight or obese by BMI; another 10 percent of the group have a normal BMI but with more body fat than is appropriate for their size. An additional 10 percent have an increased BMI but a normal proportion of body fat. It turns out that cardiovascular health as well as general quality of life, sleep quality, and brain function are not associated strictly with BMI or weight, but with the proportion of body fat relative to other tissue. So the 10 percent with a normal BMI but extra body fat appear to have health risks similar to those of their typically obese peers, a condition sometimes called normal-weight obesity. Those with a high BMI but a normal proportion of fat—generally the result of having more muscle—are no more at health risk than the totally normal person.

Although only 10 percent of the Emory Georgia Tech group was normal weight obese, some epidemiological studies indicate that the condition may be more common in Americans. Measuring body composition is more complicated than stepping on the scales, so we don't really know the extent of the problem. However, we know that the health goal is to reduce fat, and we know how to do that: diet and exercise.

By diet, we mean eating food that is, by amount and composition, appropriate for one's biology, not some distorted mix of stuff touted as the latest way to lose weight fast. One can sell a lot of books that advocate such "diets" (we are not opposed to selling books), but they are not likely to result in lasting effects on body composition. In fact, the notable failure of overweight people to lose weight and keep it off can be attributed at least in part to the virtual tsunami of fad crash diets that constantly bombards us. The word *diet* has taken on a distorted meaning to most people, and losing weight isn't the only relevant health-related outcome—indeed, as with normal-weight obesity, sometimes it's not even a reliable surrogate.

Decreasing fat and increasing lean, mostly muscle, tissue requires regular exercise as well as a prudent diet. That may be obvious, but there are also some less obvious benefits to exercise that you may not know about. Sensitivity of the body's cells to insulin, a basic abnormality in type II diabetes, improves with exercise. There is a lot of evidence that exercise helps the brain (especially executive functions). And there are even more nebulous effects on a sense of well-being, the reasons for which are not well understood. These general effects of exercise on health are likely related to effects on metabolism that are just beginning to be studied in depth.

An investigation done at Harvard measured a battery of chemicals in the blood of both poorly conditioned and well-conditioned people exercising on a treadmill, providing a picture of how their bodies were metabolizing fat, sugar, and other nutrients. Just ten minutes on the treadmill was enough to cause dramatic changes in chemicals involved in burning fat in both groups, although the changes were larger in people who were in good shape. When the researchers made similar measurements in runners who finished the 2006 Boston Marathon, the changes were ten times as great. Further, they were able to mimic the effects of exercise on muscle cells grown in culture by exposing the cells to exercise-induced chemicals; the cells' expression of genes that regulate sugar and fat metabolism was immediately increased.

We know that exercise combined with an appropriate diet will decrease body fat, thus improving health and decreasing the risk for many diseases. We are just beginning to understand some of the complexity of this effect. It is likely that there are many other effects of fat on basic body functions that await more detailed explication, which may make it possible to design diet and exercise regimens that are optimal and individual-specific.

We still have many things to learn about obesity from the biological, behavioral, and environmental angles, and even more to learn about how those factors interact. Some enticing clues are emerging. For example, some studies suggest that our individual microbiome—specifically, the bacteria that populate our intestines—can influence whether we accumulate fat and that the kind of diet we eat can affect what bacteria thrive within us. Many other novel possibilities await discovery that will no doubt open new approaches to the problem.

But making progress on the obesity problem does not have to wait for new discoveries. Many of the predictors are there, and we know what to do about them: eat right, maintain a normal proportion of body fat, exercise regularly, don't smoke cigarettes, and don't drink too much alcohol. We have the knowledge to nip this epidemic in the bud, but we haven't done it.

The fact that we know what to do and haven't done it makes obesity a great place to start to understand the opportunities of Predictive Health. We can define more clearly the complex of individual and group biology, behavior, and environment that affects why people behave badly when they know better, and we can devise healthy ways of living that are tailored to what drives each individual, including where and with whom they live. At the same time, we can start to define health in the context of the complete human experience: body, mind, and spirit. How is that complex affected by diet, exercise, biochemistry, and the perceptions and reactions of the brain/mind? What can be done about it? This epidemic is an opportunity to get a leg up on the necessary culture change—get healthy people used to engaging the system and health professionals focused on keeping people healthy.

CHAPTER 13

Evidence-Based Health

Dr. A. McGehee (Mac) Harvey was professor and chairman of the department of medicine at Johns Hopkins Hospital in the late 1960s when Mr. Hensley spent his last days there. Dr. Harvey was a taciturn Arkansan, who spoke only when he had something worthwhile to say and then in a viscous drawl typical of the region where he was born and raised. He conducted professor's rounds once a week on the Osler wards. Those rounds were occasions for residents, students, and interns to present a case to "The Professor" and then line up three deep around the patient's bed while Dr. Harvey conducted a wordless and painfully long physical examination. The cases he saw were the most difficult, those that no one could diagnose. His ability to identify even the most obscure and arcane disease was uncanny.

On one of those occasions, the patient had been in the hospital for at least a week. He had endured interminable interrogations by multiple doctors in training as well as by the best experts on the Hopkins faculty. Numerous pairs of hands had, with varying degrees of skill, poked, massaged, and prodded his fevered body. He had undergone every test that anyone could think of doing. After all that, his doctors had drawn a diagnostic blank. No one had a clue what was wrong with him . . . except The Professor.

After completing his examination, pocketing his stethoscope, and washing his hands in a bedside sink, Dr. Harvey drawled, "This patient has thrombotic thrombocytopenic purpura." Scanning the faces of his awestruck charges, he added, "Isn't that right?"

Of course as soon as Dr. Harvey massaged the available information into a diagnosis, it was perfectly obvious to even the lowliest medical student that he was correct, even if it wasn't clear why. So one red-faced medical resident blurted awkwardly, "But, Dr. Harvey, sir, what leads you to that conclusion?"

The Professor, stifling his impatience with considerable effort, answered, "What else could it be?"

Medicine for Dr. Harvey did not appear to be an intellectual exercise in the usual sense. He didn't appear to sort through any logical decision tree (or if he did, he certainly didn't communicate that to his students). Diagnosis for him seemed to be an intuitive process of fitting a body of information into a pattern and comparing it to the thousands of mental templates he had accumulated over years of experience. If he knew how he arrived at a diagnostic conclusion (one suspects that he didn't, at least in any analytical way), he was either unable or unwilling to explain it to anyone else. He didn't deal in differential diagnoses, the prioritized list of possibilities in a given case. He didn't deal in statistical probabilities. To him the diagnosis was obvious. What else could it be?

The Professor's method may sound decidedly unscientific, but it may surprise you to know that evidence-based medicine as currently practiced is a relatively recent concept (for practical purposes dating to Archie Cochrane's 1972 book, *Effectiveness and Efficiency: Random Reflections on Health Services,* and first named by Gordon Guyatt in a 1992 article in the *Journal of the American Medical Association*). The practice of medicine, even for most of the modern era, has largely been an exercise in intuition informed by experience and knowledge, using pattern recognition more than critical analysis.

That was the only way to do it when accessing the ever-proliferating medical literature was laborious and time consuming, involving card catalogs, the Dewey Decimal System, *Current Contents*, and the *Index Medicus*—which now seem quaint and ludicrously clumsy attempts to make entrée into collective knowledge. Even the biggest and most facile brain could not retain each individual bit of the information, and there was neither time nor energy to search it out. The answer to this dilemma for creative brains was to piece together individual bits of information into patterns, like solving a jigsaw puzzle, and then to remember the pattern. Dr. Harvey was one of a few who were extraordinarily good at retaining and recalling those patterns.

The advent of the information age changed everything, putting virtually the entire repository of human knowledge, much of it already analyzed and presented as "best practices," in a handheld computer. There are no longer any legendary clinicians, their uncanny clinical insight elevating them head and shoulders above their peers. Everyone has the same information. The playing field is level. The medical world is flat.

Well, not exactly. It is easy to agree that the best scientific evidence should drive how doctors diagnose and treat sick people, but implementing that idea is not so simple. As often as not, the best evidence is inconclusive; in 2007, 49 percent of 1,016 reviews of various treatments by the Cochrane Collaborations Review Groups (the accepted authorities) found that the treatments were neither clearly beneficial nor clearly harmful, and 96 percent recommended more research on the reviewed topic. In plain English, it's hard to reduce medical practice to a universally applicable decision tree—often the evidence is just not there, and something has to be done anyway. Also, many practicing doctors don't buy it. Some see the whole idea of evidence-based medicine as a conspiracy of managers to infringe on their independence for the sole purpose of saving money. Others think that there is just no substitute for clinical judgment, the nebulous, idiosyncratic experience of the lone practitioner on the front lines interacting with the individual patient, things that are difficult to codify and enter into a database.

But even if you buy the concept, what is credible evidence? One attempt to codify credibility involves defining a hierarchy of evidence. Level I evidence, under this scheme the most credible, requires well-designed, randomized, controlled clinical trials, with the results appearing in a reputable journal that requires review and acceptance by a panel of the authors' peers in order to be published. Levels II-1, II-2, and II-3 include studies of decreasing scientific rigor, and level III includes the "opinions of respected authorities based on clinical experience, descriptive studies, or reports of committees."

But even the most expert review of available evidence using this or some other assessment of credibility can't escape the fact that about half of what is done in medicine must be done without clear evidence one way or the other. David Sackett, professor of medicine at Oxford (and one of the progenitors of this approach), argues that evidence-based medicine is "about integrating individual clinical experience and the best external evidence." Apparently Dr. Sackett would not exclude clinicians of Dr. Harvey's ilk as a resource. Try as we might to make medical practice a strict science, a need for the art of medicine persists.

Experience is also a source of evidence; practice-based evidence should be a critical part of evidence-based practice. If we could know the outcomes of a given intervention in a given situation for every doctor, say in the United States or even the entire world, that should help with the answers to the questions that evidence-based medicine seeks. Does a treatment work? What are the details of the situations in which it does or doesn't? If that information were available electronically, then any physician's patient could benefit from the collective experience of the whole profession with a particular condition and its possible treatments. And the body of information would be dynamic; each new incident of treatment would expand the available evidence for or against it. This is of course an ideal, and as our discussion of health records shows, all of the pieces are not in place yet. But some are, and more are on the way.

At its best, then, medical care would integrate scientific evidence, the collective clinical experience, and insight from superior clinicians gained by their personal experience, to take the best care of each person needing it. We suspect that medicine will remain both an art and a science.

Although Predictive Health focuses on health instead of disease, it shares goals with the practice of medicine: Evidence, experience, and insight must support practices. Given how far we are from understanding and defining health and unhealth, the distance to cover to reach those goals for health-focused care is an order of magnitude greater than for evidence-based medicine.

The issue of evidence in Predictive Health involves more than medical practitioners and their teachers. A large, health-targeted industry has developed that is as easy to access as the vitamin store in the nearest strip mall. A range of practices and products, commonly lumped together as complementary and alternative medicine, and a developing field of integrative medicine use these approaches in addition to allopathic (that is, conventional) medicine.

This burgeoning health-targeted industry concerns us, especially the vigorous marketing of highly profitable products that are often short on evidence of either effectiveness or safety. Chains of shops with row on row of vitamins, herbs, and extracts of various plants and animals—with sales rivaling those of the entire pharmaceutical industry—thrive, supported by an abundance of myths, often perpetuated uncritically by people who are otherwise perfectly rational. Let's look at a few examples of things meant to maintain or improve health.

The term *nutraceuticals* was coined by Stephen DeFelice to refer to things derived from food that have an assumed or proven health benefit and are either added to foods or taken as a supplement to them. This includes the iodine added to salt, vitamin D added to milk, folic acid added to flour, as well as beta-carotene, lycopene, alpha-lipoic acid, and other popular pills and capsules. Close to two-thirds of Americans take at least one of these products, and the industry as a whole has annual sales of some $86 billion, luring even the big pharmaceutical firms (e.g., DuPont, Abbot Laboratories, Johnson & Johnson, and Novartis) into the act.

Reasonable evidence supports the effectiveness of a number of nutraceuticals with specific targets, but many products are marketed as having health benefits—like preventing chronic diseases, delaying aging, or increasing longevity—when there is absolutely no objective reason to think they can do those things. The marketers may put a disclaimer in the fine print (such as "there is no scientific proof for the claims made on the label"), but the headlines promise all kinds of outrageous results. What's worse, there is essentially no accountability for false claims. A field day for marketers. Not so good for the unwary seeker of youth and immortality. But, that is where our society has decided responsibility must lie. If you choose to take dietary supplements, some due diligence is in order, and you will have to do it for yourself. (A good place to start is to remember that things that seem too good to be true usually are.)

In chapter 5 we discussed the difficulties in proving that any given component of a food is either safe or effective when taken out of context, separated from the complex mixture in which one ordinarily consumes it. Given the complexity of biology, it is likely that interactions of ingredients in a healthy diet are essential for positive effects. The concept of *functional foods* captures the idea that whole foods may have favorable effects that exceed their apparent nutritional value. This concept may help explain things like the Mediterranean diet phenomenon where interactions of foods taken together may have positive health effects that no single component of the diet consumed in the same quantities in isolation has.

Homeopathy is a historically durable system of treatments based on the idea that something that may be toxic can have positive health effects if diluted enough and shaken vigorously with each dilution (a process called succussion). Often the dilutions are so great that there is no possibility that any of the original substance is still there. The entire concept seems absurd on its surface. However, dismissing homeopathy as silly is complicated by published studies in highly reputable journals by some eminent scientists making claims that seem to support the general idea. A now notorious article by Jacques Beneviste in the elite scientific journal *Nature* in 1988 claimed that human antibodies continued to have activity in solutions so dilute that they could not possibly have contained any antibodies. And none other than the French Nobel Prize winner Luc Montagnier (a codiscoverer of the AIDS virus) recently claimed that a dilute solution of DNA could send electromagnetic imprints from one test tube (through two glass walls) to an adjacent one containing only water and the DNA replicated in the tube with only water. There are also some clinical studies. One such study, published in the journal *Chest*, reports that a solution of potassium dichromate, diluted so much that there would remain only one molecule in a sphere with a diameter equal to the distance from the earth to the sun (not our calculation), had a positive effect on lung function in patients in intensive care units. To say that such observations stretch credulity is a serious understatement.

The clinical practice of homeopathy has a long history and continues, with even some very smart scientists still entranced by the wonder of it all. There are many who believe, and they can cite personal experience, that homeopathic interventions work. The operative word may be *believe.* Virtually all of the careful reviews of available evidence conclude that such treatments are no different than the effects of placebos, that is, inert treatments like sugar pills or sham surgeries. The Latin root of the term *placebo* means, "I shall please." There is power, biological power, in being told by a credible authority that some intervention is active and is expected to have a positive effect. Placebos do often work, in the sense that they have a biological effect that mimics the effect of an active intervention to which they are compared. *The Powerful Placebo*, published in 1955 by Henry Beecher, makes the point that such interventions may even have clinically important effects. Whether such effects actually require administering the placebo or are just a consequence of the Hawthorne effect (that is, people will report feeling better just because they know they are being studied to see if they do feel better) is debatable. A *Cochrane Review* published in 2010 suggested the Hawthorne effect as the explanation. There is continuing discussion about whether placebos are useful as therapy and whether the necessary deception is ethical. Placebos seem to be stuck between the Scylla of empiricism and the Charybdis of scientific rigor. Or, if you prefer a terrestrial metaphor, between a rock and a hard place.

Increasingly popular mind-body practices also deserve scrutiny. Meditation, long a core practice of Eastern religions, is now a common part of health-focused behaviors in this country. Until recently the evidence that it worked (that is, had any effects on biology) was largely from personal testimonials and the centuries-long Eastern experience. But recently objective and scientifically sound investigations have convinced even a lot of serious skeptics that there are biologic effects of meditation, that (as many of us suspected all along) the head bone is connected to the body bone. It certainly makes intuitive and experiential sense that what goes on in the brain (thoughts, fantasies, emotions, deceptions, schemes, calculations, sensations) can have an effect on biologically measurable functions of the body. Those connections are potentially manageable and could be prime targets for Predictive Health.

Some powerful evidence for positive effects of meditation has been produced by Chuck Raison, a sandy haired ex-Californian and pleasantly rumpled, middle-aged psychiatrist, who was formerly a member of the Emory faculty. Raison has made a career out of this mind-body connection, with a focus on compassion meditation as practiced by Buddhists such as the Dalai Lama, who is himself a member of the visiting Emory faculty. Dr. Raison and his colleagues set about to bring some scientific rigor to evaluating the practice. In one study done with a group of college students, they determined the effects of compassion meditation on the body's response to psychosocial stress.

This kind of research employs a standardized (and interesting) way to create psychosocial stress in an experimental setting. It even works in college students. The test is a contrived scene in which the subject is given a brief time to prepare a speech on a given topic. The subject then delivers the speech before a panel of "judges," whose stern faces betray nothing about how they are reacting to the performance. The results are striking. Subjects get nervous. They sweat. Their faces flush. Their blood pressure goes up. Their pulses race. And the amounts of several chemicals in the blood that indicate inflammation go way up. In short, the body responds to psychosocial stress much as it responds to infection with a virus or a bacterium.

Raison had two groups of students, matched as well as possible. Both groups were required to participate in twelve hours of classes. In one group, these classes were sessions of compassion meditation presented as a secular (nonreligious) exercise but based on an ancient Tibetan Buddhist practice called *lojong*. The other (control) group had classes on topics relevant to the mental and physical health of college students but no meditation. Both groups were given a compact disc to aid them in continuing the experience at home. At the end of the twelve-week study, when the stress tests were done, the meditators did indeed have significantly less evidence of stress and significantly less inflammation, and—here is the interesting part—the effect was dose related. The high-practice meditating group had significantly greater reduction in the stress response than the students in the control group, but also greater than the low-practice meditators. In short, the response pattern was like that usually seen with drugs. Dr. Raison and his friends have a grant from the National Institutes of Health to extend these studies to other groups of people and to increase the rigor of the experimental design, meaning that it is too early to claim that they have unequivocally proved a beneficial physical effect of meditation. But it isn't too early to imagine how this work could have profound implications. Most of the major chronic human diseases—heart disease, diabetes, Alzheimer's disease, maybe even depression—are associated with chronic inflammation. A means of fixing a fundamental mechanism, well before disease develops—the core of our health-focused approach—that requires no special equipment or gym membership and is affordable by everyone, would be an intensely exciting development.

Accumulating the knowledge available about the myriad things people do and take in an effort to stay healthy, analyzing it objectively, and making it readily available—implementing the concept of evidence-based health with the same energy, passion, and resources being spent on evidence-based medicine—would be a major advance. Realizing the goal of Predictive Health will require everything available—diet, exercise, supplements, yoga, meditation—whatever works and is safe. But as with things used to diagnose and treat disease, we have to continue to insist on developing the best possible evidence. Otherwise we are wasting time, effort, and money and likely taking unnecessary risks. Predictive Health is a powerful idea with the potential to radically change how we go about ensuring our health and well-being, but without evidence it is only a sterile intellectual exercise or a seductive ideology.

CHAPTER 14

Good Drugs

Making Health Pills

A FEW YEARS AGO Emory University hosted Futurist Forum, a panel of fifteen of the country's foremost thought leaders, to discuss future trends in the study of the social, physical, and biological sciences. The moderator of the panel was Stephen Frazier, at the time a popular CNN news anchor. Mr. Frazier was an attractive, well-dressed, slightly overweight, middle-aged guy. His performance that morning was impressively articulate and strikingly perceptive, but even before the program began he demonstrated the aplomb with which he would lead the discussion when he was lured into a conversation about Predictive Health.

The question was how, under Predictive Health, we would get people to do what they need to do to stay healthy. Our response, the Predictive Health mantra, was that we would engage people in a partnership that focuses on healthy life choices, give them the information they need, and help with the strategy and support the tactics necessary to do something useful with it.

"Come on," Mr. Frazier responded. "This is America. It will have to be a pill."

He made an important point. We love pills and either take or seek them for almost everything—weight loss, libido, moodiness, insomnia, lethargy, nebulous aches and pains, even aging, as though aging were a disease to be cured. We are a nation of pillophiles.

Doctors also love pills. We prescribe them at the slightest hint of some possible effect, nurturing the expectation that they will work. We make pills so readily available that we are probably abusing them both as patients and as doctors. But that is the culture we are in, and it's not likely to change anytime soon. So we might as well try to take advantage of the situation and seek new pills with health rather than disease as their target.

Unencumbered by a need for very much rigorous scientific evidence, the hucksters are ahead of us here. *Life Extension* magazine, published by the eponymous Life Extension Foundation, lists the top ten most popular "life extension" drugs. The list includes synthetic human growth hormone—and the contact information for a doctor who will prescribe it for between $12,000 and $225,000 per year (we suppose the lawyers do have to be paid)—as well as melatonin, which the magazine claims might "possibly protect us against every age-related disease known to mankind" (the hedging betrays the claim's bald absurdity) and is available from the Life Extension Buyers Club.

But wait, there's more! One company sells a pill containing the extract of a freshwater algae said to exist in only one place in the world (at the bottom of Oregon's Klamath Lake) to "maintain healthy stem cell physiology." There is a whole list of so-called immune-enhancing pills, one for example containing a chemical found in broccoli and some other vegetables, said to be "a potent activator of the immune response system," that is taken every day by fifteen Nobel Prize winners and five thousand physicians. Kava kava, pygeum, bonge oil, dong quai, piracetum, GH3/KH3, centrophenoxine—the range of options is very large, exceeded only by the magnitude of the accompanying claims.

Our skepticism is obvious, and deliberately so. It rests on our respect for science and our collective century of experience in medicine and health care. It is true that empiricism has served the field of medicine well in many cases and continues to do so. Where understanding of human health and disease is incomplete, we necessarily rely on experience and best rationale. But that cannot be used to sanction the unregulated marketing of pills making global health claims that are unproven or even unprovable. Panaceas burst on the scene from time to time with great fanfare, only to slink away after a brief spell of fame into oblivion, their metaphorical tails tucked ashamedly between their legs, having done little good and sometimes great harm. Someone will always be ready to aggressively sell anything that people will try. Things that sound too good to be true usually are—caveat emptor—but that doesn't mean that we couldn't, despite the quackery, make pills to enhance health rather than treat disease.

The conventional course of drug discovery goes something like this: 1) pick a process (chemical reaction, cell response) that you want to affect, 2) create a system to measure the target process in thousands of samples very quickly, 3) acquire a group (library) of thousands of chemical compounds (they are commercially available), 4) determine which of these compounds affect your target process (these are called hits), 5) analyze each of the hits closely to be sure they are having the effect, 6) test for safety and efficacy in animals, 7) test for safety in normal humans, and 8) test for safety and efficacy in humans with the disease you intend to treat.

The process may sound simple, but it's not. For good reasons, this is an expensive, time-consuming, complex, and highly regulated process. The following figure illustrates two of the challenges. One is the time it takes to get from initial screening of possible agents to completing clinical trials and seeking approval to market from the FDA—six and one-half years from initial screening to the very first trials in humans and an additional eight and one-half years to finish development: a total of fifteen years. The second challenge is the

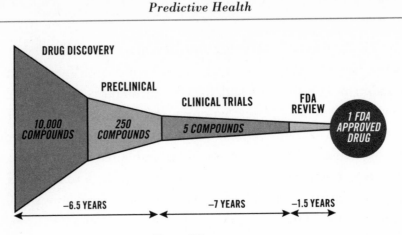

DRUG DISCOVERY

PRECLINICAL

CLINICAL TRIALS

FDA REVIEW

10,000 COMPOUNDS

250 COMPOUNDS

5 COMPOUNDS

1 FDA APPROVED DRUG

−6.5 YEARS   −7 YEARS   −1.5 YEARS

Drug Discovery

winnowing process, finding the one candidate agent in ten thousand possibilities that can clear all of the necessary developmental hurdles, the safe and effective needle in the haystack of toxins, placebos, and duds. Then there is the cost; estimates are that it costs almost $2 billion to develop a drug from start to finish. Regulation adds to both the time and dollar costs of drug development, but we think—despite the occasional call for revising and reducing it—this is necessary. And despite the hurdles, researchers are working to discover drugs that promote health through the accepted development process.

One target has been the regenerative potential of stem cells. In fact, the algal extract discussed previously seems to temporarily increase the number of stem cells circulating in blood, a possible indicator of the vigor of the regenerative process. There are several other drugs on the market that do the same thing; their primary use is collecting donor cells for a stem cell transplant—a common treatment for some life-threatening diseases for several years now.

But a drug of this sort, meant to enhance health, would have to clear some significant hurdles in the standard drug development scenario. First, there are several different breeds of stem cells that may do different things, and effects on the kind and number of these cells would have to be shown. Second, investigators would have to show that increasing stem-cell circulation in essentially healthy people actually makes them healthier. A producer of plant extracts like the Oregon algae pill can already make such claims because the FDA can't regulate such products. For a regulated drug to make claims like that, it would have to be shown that the specific kind of stem cell that the drug increased affected something that everyone agreed indicated improved health (such as improved function of blood vessels). Finally, and very important, this drug mustn't make healthy people sick. There would be very little tolerance for any bad side effects (a burden not borne by the plant extract manufacturers).

Sometimes researchers get lucky during the drug screening process and find a shortcut around some of the hurdles. This was the case for Leonard Zon and his colleagues at Children's Hospital Boston, who are looking for drugs to affect stem cells. They were screening drugs in special zebra fish, tiny, transparent fish that absorb chemicals through their skin, to see what effects a panel of drugs had on circulating stem cells. This approach usually identifies a large number of hits, which must be winnowed to find the most effective and least toxic candidate. That can require hundreds of studies in animals and cells before one is ready for human trials, but Zon and his colleagues were lucky. Their big hit was with a drug that was already being given to humans for other reasons, enabling them to skip directly to a first phase of human trials. If the drug does ultimately prove successful, they're only eight years from the finish line.

Another target of health-focused drug research has been a drug that mimics exercise—exactly where Stephen Frazier said we should focus. Ron Evans and his colleagues at the Salk Institute reported in 2008 the discovery of two drugs that affected metabolism in mouse muscle cells just like exercise.

Four years before that announcement, Evans and his friends had begun their work using genetic engineering to create a "marathon mouse" by altering a gene, called PPAR-delta, known to be involved in physical conditioning. The modified mice stayed thin, had low amounts of fat in their blood, and had low blood sugar regardless of their diets. What's more, they could run on a mouse treadmill twice as far as normal mice. These mice, thanks to their engineered version of this gene, were inherently fit. The researchers then investigated a list of drugs with known effects on PPAR to see if they could find a drug with this same effect. They did. Medicated mice increased fat burning, decreased blood sugar, increased exercise capacity, and looked for all the world just as fit (in some cases more so) as mice that had been for weeks on a rigorous exercise program. Not surprising that Dr. Oz, Oprah, and the *Wall Street Journal* went gaga. (An amusing piece in the August 1, 2008, *Wall Street Journal* by Peter Jeffrey imagines an interesting year 2025 in which drugs like these are widely available.)

Dr. Evans himself wasn't shy about speculating on the implications. "We have now created the potential for a really simple intervention in the area of major health problems for which there is no intervention," he said, adding that it could be perfect for people who wanted the benefits of exercise without the work. Heady speculation, indeed, but there is a ways to go to get to a pill that will replace exercise in healthy people. The likelihood of either of these drugs ending up in history's dustbin is not small; the path to success is tortuous, complex, and expensive. What keeps researchers and pharmaceutical companies going this direction is both the thrill of discovery and some very tangible possible future rewards. Remember that Americans spend $86 billion a year on nutraceuticals alone. That kind of market could easily justify scientific development of health pills—the market appeal of proven agents ought to easily outstrip the appeal of those based on sheer hype. Surely, given the option, any consumer will find substance more convincing than style.

The case file for health-directed pills already contains at least one precedent—statins, taken by tens of millions of Americans every day. Statins are a class of drugs that were developed in the standard way by major pharmaceutical companies to lower the amount of cholesterol in the blood and so decrease the risk of a heart attack, presumably even in people who have never had a heart attack or any other indication that there is anything wrong with their heart and circulation. They just have high cholesterol. So these are essentially healthy people being given a drug to make them healthier. Even in this success story, there is, however, a cautionary tale. Statins do have side effects; some minor side effects were found before the drugs were approved for mass marketing, but some seem to show up only after prolonged use. That illustrates the clear dilemma for health pills: We want to use only safe ones, but in some cases we can't know they are completely safe until they have been taken for much longer than is practical for the typical drug trial. But when compared to the minimally regulated marketing of plant-derived supplements with elaborate claims, unproven effect, and unknown toxicity, this approach to developing drugs that make people healthier still has appeal.

Even if we had well-tested health pills, probably not everyone would need to take them. Mr. Hensley didn't do very well in the lifestyle department, and he paid dearly for that with a good portion of his potential life. If he could have taken pills that made him fit and endowed him with the stem cells of a youth, he might have done that and lived a lot longer and healthier. But Ms. Echt did pretty well for over a century. Maybe she didn't need the pills.

CHAPTER 15

Disrupting Medical Care

Realizing Predictive Health

MEDICAL CARE IS preoccupied with disease. People do not usually go to see a doctor unless they are sick. And doctors are not very interested in people who are well. It is the fascinating cases—"fascinomas" in medical student lingo—that mesmerize them. Has a conversation among doctors (or health-care professionals of any stripe) ever included someone exulting over the experience of caring for a totally healthy person? No. It is always disease that dominates those conversations. People are often defined by their disease (the cystic fibrotic, the hypertensive, the diabetic), or even equated to it (the meningitis up on 2C). That has to change, or we will not get healthier, and we will go broke in the process. Our culture must move beyond medicine as we have known it.

Beyond medicine to what? To a health-focused system that captures the attention (and imagination) of healthy people and of those charged with participating in their care. To a system that values a sense of wonder and curiosity about each incredible human being. To a system that understands our biological, emotional, and spiritual selves and learns to integrate those into an identity that is happy and productive—that flourishes.

Creating a health-care system that focuses on health will require some major education on all sides. We need a new vocabulary, new kinds of physical facilities (spare us the antiseptic smell of pale green, cookie cutter doctors' offices with pictures of men in red coats riding to hounds), new kinds of health-care providers, and new social attitudes. In short, we need to change the culture. And most of all we need to feel and share the ecstasy of discovering our healthy selves.

Predictive Health is about better science and a better understanding of our position at the intersection of biology, behavior, and environment. But it is more than that, and to succeed, it must change the game, and not just by replacing the obsession with fighting disease with an emphasis on defining and preserving health. Predictive Health aims to disrupt everything you and the medical community know about health care. It can do that given the right groundwork. Indeed, given the right groundwork, disruption is not just possible, it's inevitable.

Disruption isn't just about having potent knowledge; it is about applying that knowledge. Consider the history of the computer in science. In the early 1970s using a computer in scientific research involved huge stacks of punch cards, long waits for access to a mainframe machine, and the help of multiple experts. Over the ensuing decades, something major changed—computing, the exclusive domain of a priestly class, became easy to use and relatively inexpensive, and access was democratized. Science was disrupted as a result.

Clayton Christensen and his colleagues at the Harvard Business School and Innosight, LLC have written at some length about disruptive innovations in health care in books and journal articles. Disruptive innovations are not just powerful—they are accessible and cheap, which is why they disrupt. Considering medicine, Christensen, in *The Innovator's Prescription*, argues that rather than relying on "complex, high-cost institutions and expensive, specialized professionals," we should, "move down-market . . . look at the problem in a very different way . . . [and] focus instead on enabling less expensive professionals to do progressively more sophisticated things in less expensive settings"—very much like the way the personal computer enables science to be done in situations impossible during the heyday of the mainframe. Christensen's book deals mostly with improved diagnosis and treatment, with patients, not people, but we think we can extend his point to ours, including his discussion of opposition to innovation by entrenched interests. And if the disruption of innovation in medical care threatens the myriad constituencies who sup generously from the current medical care trough, Predictive Health is another level of threat.

Predictive Health needs more than just new knowledge to realize its potential to disrupt. We have covered here much of the necessary science, but have only alluded to some of the cultural implications. A primary need is for a new mindset; measurements are not made to establish a diagnosis but to define the status of a person's health. Predictions based on data are not of risk for a heart attack or Alzheimer's disease, but the odds of staying healthy. And that new mindset requires a new vocabulary. Words and how we use them matter. People are people, not patients. Healthy people encountering the care system should neither perceive themselves as patients nor be perceived that way by care providers. They must be understood as real human beings, with all of the marvelous potential that that implies, and our job as health-care professionals is to help them see that potential and go about realizing it.

Predictive Health also needs new facilities—not just new hospitals or clinics, but novel places that look, feel, and function differently than anything in the current system. Built environments matter. They affect the health and well-being of the human beings who encounter them. The entire discipline of architecture is based on that fundamental concept. So these new places would be real health-care facilities, welcoming and engaging spaces that healthy people seek out to learn about their health and to discover how to stay as healthy as they can be; they must not be repositories of the sick and maimed.

Predictive Health requires the integration of health and well-being. Contemporary medicine draws a fairly bright line separating the objective biology from the more subjective sense of well-being. When doctors fail to identify a physical cause for a patient's complaints, they lose interest, often labeling the patient as a hypochondriac or (informally) a croc (for chronic complainer). The labels are pejorative and result in complaints being dismissed with a curt, "it's in your head," as though psyche and soma lived in different spaces. Subjectivity is not a favored approach to understanding human misery among doctors trained to honor objective science. Medical doctors are proud to live and work with only the biology, perfectly happy to cede the other territories to their less rigorous colleagues.

When Mr. Hensley was admitted to the Johns Hopkins Hospital in 1966, he got the best medical care available anywhere at the time. Probably none of the cadre of elite health professionals who cared for him bothered to ask him or his devoted wife how he felt about his life, whether he was troubled, afraid, or felt fulfilled, or what things brought him pleasure and made him happy. It may not have mattered much at the end, but it is likely that during his entire life not a single encounter with the health-care system had elicited that kind of information—and earlier, before he was dying, such information may have made a difference. Had the system paid more attention to the environments and behaviors that so profoundly affected his biology, he may have taken a different course, relied less on alcohol and paid more attention to caring for his diabetes. In fact, part of the contrasting lives of Mr. Hensley and Ms. Echt likely had something to do with how much attention they each paid to the subjectivity of the life experience.

Subjective well-being is a topic of serious research. The methods are different than biologists use, but there is rigor in the effort. University of Illinois psychologist Ed Diener and colleagues define subjective well-being as, "the scientific analysis of how people evaluate their lives." They aim to understand the role of well-being in the quality of life of individual people and societies. But like medical doctors, researchers in this area tend to work in their own fields and think in their own paradigms, failing to integrate biology and well-being.

There are some signs that the disruption we predict is already underway. Some years ago, Penny George had cancer. Her medical doctors went diligently about trying to rid her body of the malignant cells without doing more harm than was necessary. But she needed something more. Facing cancer is more than dealing with a glob of malignant cells. More than a disease of the body, cancer is a disease of the head, the heart, and the soul. So Dr. George, a psychologist, investigated complementary approaches to healing that paid more attention to the whole experience. Chemotherapy and whatever else modern oncology had to offer eradicated the malignant cells. Complementary interventions wrested her heart and soul from the threat of cancer's grasp. Her cancer was cured.

Penny George was determined to spread the word. She and her husband (Bill is a professor at Harvard Business School and former CEO of Medtronics) established the Penny George Institute for Health and Healing in Minneapolis. But they went further. They created the Bravewell Collaborative, a collection of people and initiatives, including integrative medicine programs in academic institutions across the country, that deal with people as whole people: mind, body, and spirit. Their facilities, vocabulary, and approach bring something new and different to health care, complementing the best of science and technology with time-tested alternative methods. When Penny George shows you around the Minneapolis facility, her elegant professional façade softens. She smiles a lot. She must be proud of what she has created; she certainly should be.

There are other examples. The Duke Center for Integrative Medicine lives (thanks to an $11 million gift from the Christy and John Mack Foundation) in a beautiful, freestanding facility designed by Duda/Paine Architects that is a bold physical expression of the integrative medicine concept. The Scripps Center for Integrative Medicine has the distinct esthetic advantage of a spectacular view of the Pacific Ocean from many parts of the facility. These and several other programs pay attention to the integration of biology, environment, and behavior as essential to health and well-being.

All of these facilities, however, are not practicing Predictive Health—they all have a major focus on treating disease. For an even more disruptive experience, visit the eighteenth floor of Emory University Midtown Hospital in Atlanta, home of the Emory Georgia Tech Center for Health Discovery and Well Being,® where we work. Unlike those other facilities, this one deals only with essentially healthy people. You don't come here to see a doctor. You don't need symptoms to be welcome here. This is Predictive Health in action.

First-time visitors—we call them "participants," not patients—undergo a battery of the latest biological tests, including measures of body fat, bone density, circulatory function, inflammatory status, physical fitness, and brain function. The four fundamental processes—immune function, inflammation, oxidative stress, and regenerative capacity—are charted, and samples of blood are biobanked. All of that information, plus extensive information about the person's environment and behaviors, is compiled into a health assessment report, and a health action plan is developed. Each participant goes through all this with a "Predictive Health partner," a new, key professional who accompanies each participant on the quest for optimal health.

It's too early to tell conclusively what the results of this program are, but there are some encouraging signs. As of March 2011, the center had enrolled slightly more than seven hundred people. Except for a few paying customers, these are a random sample of Emory University's twenty thousand or so employees (paid for by a grant from the Cousins Foundation and by the institution as a proof of concept). We sought them out. They didn't come because they were looking for help with their health. In spite of that, the majority of those who completed the initial evaluation have stuck with the program, returning for their repeat evaluations at six months and then annually. Many of the participants hadn't paid much attention to their health before this. Maybe getting people engaged has an effect.

Certainly the participants seem to be getting healthier, with marked improvements after six months for the first three hundred or so participants. For the group as a whole, a lot of things got better, and some were unexpected, certainly in so short a time. Biology improved: weight decreased, blood pressure went down, blood sugar decreased, blood lipids improved, biomarkers of inflammation got better. The surprises came in measures of well-being, although if we really believed what we said about the interdependence of physical health and well-being, perhaps they shouldn't have been surprises: perceived stress decreased, quality of life was better, and there was less depression.

That's what happened in the group as a whole, regardless of what the individual opportunities were at the start. Some of the individual stories are even more impressive. A high-ranking elected official enrolled in the program and lost about forty pounds over a year. When asked what about the program motivated him, he said without hesitating that it was the health partner. He gave her his cell phone number, and she kept in touch. He said he felt responsible to her. We suppose that responsible behavior in relationships is important to politicians.

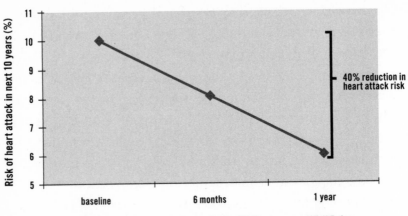

Effect of Participation in Center for Health Discovery
and Well Being on Risk for Heart Attack

An aging physician participant started out in pretty good health. He said he exercised fairly regularly and watched what he ate. He felt that he was healthy. But he learned some things he didn't know about his health and worked with a health partner to make a plan. In a year (see the graph), his heart attack risk decreased by 40 percent.

An executive's wife had marked improvement in a number of areas after only six months in the program. She said that her motivator was the body scan, which screens for body composition, including body fat. For most of us, viewing a graphic picture of our body fat is not a pleasant experience. It can be motivating.

Whether these individual and group effects last, only time will tell. And we will need more time and deeper analysis of the data to know exactly why they happen. However, things certainly look promising so far.

The center's information bank is also revealing things we didn't know about human health. As others have suggested and we discussed earlier, BMI is not as accurate a measure of obesity as generally thought; we're extending this idea to determine precisely how percent body fat relates to BMI and how obesity (by either measure) is influenced by biology, behavior, and environment. We found that vitamin D deficiency is common in our participants, and the amount of that vitamin measured in the blood correlates with many measures of cardiovascular and metabolic health. Early results indicate that for participants whose vitamin D levels increased between their initial visit and their revisit at six months, cardiovascular health improved. Cardiovascular health didn't improve in participants whose D levels stayed low. But it's early yet, and there is much more to be discovered. Investigators are using the center data and biobanked samples to explore how sleep patterns, nutrition, meditation, gene expression, metabolomic profile, and a variety of other factors relate to health. Center participants will be the first to benefit from new discoveries.

Participants also get some fringe benefits. Although the center and its health partners do not practice medicine, participants discovered to need medical care are directed to the appropriate professionals. There are some examples of information making a dramatic difference. Serum hormone levels led to the diagnosis and treatment of a benign tumor of the pituitary gland. An unsuspected irregular pulse led to diagnosis and treatment of a potentially serious heart condition. Numerous participants with unsuspected high blood pressure, diabetes, high cholesterol, and more have been channeled to the right place for medical care. These were people who didn't come to the center for diagnosis and treatment. Their conditions would likely have continued untreated for much longer if not for the program.

More must change for approaches like this to become mainstream—health care must cease to be top-down. All these innovative programs are top-down in the sense that they all rely on philanthropy. The dollars have come from the George, Mack, and

Cousins Foundations (and there are undoubtedly numerous other philanthropic gifts that have made such programs possible) and commitments from forward-thinking institutions that care about health and also understand the academic opportunity. Our current healthcare system doesn't pay for most of this, certainly not for the programs that focus on keeping people healthy. A few interested people are having a go at it, but the total number of people benefiting from these innovative programs is minuscule compared to the country's population. We expect there will be an opportunity to change that, to disrupt the status quo, as the word gets out. People will demand it. For that to happen, Predictive Health needs to go viral.

Already upward of two-thirds of adult Americans look online for health information, and over half say what they found out changed how they approached their own health or that of someone for whom they cared. Though this may not be the domain of MySpace, Facebook, and Twitter, where users don't talk much about health, there are other indications that information and social experience in the cyberworld are grasping the health opportunity.

There is an interminable list of Web sites that provide information and advice about diseases or assemble affinity groups who have or have survived health challenges (often cancer). Dailystrength.org, for example, enables discussions among patients and caregivers of hundreds of medical issues, provides support communities, accesses information, and even lets users send a virtual hug. The CDC and the American Cancer Society are experimenting with the cyberworld as a way to affect attitudes about nutrition, cancer screening, and infectious disease risk. There is even a Mayo Clinic Center for Social Media, which hosts the Social Media Health Network, providing the means for combining social media and health care. If you want to start something in cyberspace, you can call on the expertise of that venerable institution for help.

Social networking as a way to change the culture of health is especially attractive because of the target demographic. Although old dogs may be able—with enough effort and assistance—to learn a new trick or two, it's a lot easier for the young. Culture change is a future-directed effort. It doesn't happen at warp speed. Get the teens on board, and you have a chance to do something really big. Presumably with that in mind, the Institute of Medicine and the National Academy of Engineering launched a program called Go Viral to Improve Health. The initiative challenges college and university students to build apps using the organizations' data to address pressing health issues, to "engage and empower people in ways that lead to better health." This just might have a chance of doing something interesting since it engages the same people you want to excite in the process of generating the excitement, makes the customer the salesman.

There is more to such exercises than may be apparent. While health is ultimately a personal issue, it cannot be separated from social experience. For example, a thirty-two-year study of twelve thousand people published in 2007 concluded that friends, siblings, and spouses have a greater effect on an individual's risk for obesity than genetics. It will take more than a village to make us as healthy as we can be; it will take a vast network of villages. The networks are there. They are changing culture in many ways at a speed not possible until recently. The technology continues to expand, as do the possibilities.

A major challenge for Predictive Health is training the professionals to provide it. Just as these organizations cannot rely solely on philanthropy for long-term survival, they cannot rely solely on educating their employees after the fact, after the medical education establishment has done its disease-centric work. Predictive Health must have people trained for the job, which means that the education of physicians must change, and new roles must be defined and filled. A focus on health must permeate the education of health-care professionals at all levels. Predictive Health, of course, will not eliminate disease or injury, but those things should cease to be the sole focus of professional education. Rather, physiology, normal structure and function, should dominate pathology in the curricula. Understanding how things go right should trump understanding what happens when things go wrong.

There is more to Christensen's picture of a disruptive medical technology that will enable "less expensive professionals to do progressively more sophisticated things in less expensive settings." Predictive Health will require heeding his advice. The numbers don't work otherwise. Caring for healthy people increases the denominator a lot (there are many more well people than sick ones), so just expanding the responsibilities of current health professionals is not feasible. It doesn't make sense anyway to have highly trained, expensive professionals operating way below their level of competence. They are not happy with that arrangement; they cost too much and probably do those tasks less well than people trained specifically to do them. There are also issues about what is done and how, as well as who does it and where.

A criticism of modern medicine is what has been called overdiagnosis, the idea that the more tests we have done, the more likely we are to be pronounced ill. Predictive Health's answer to this critique is to change the mindset of health-care workers. If they are trained to diagnose—to find sickness—they will do that. But if their orientation is to understand and address health, they should not contribute to the overdiagnosis problem. The problem is not that we are measuring too many things, but that we are measuring too few (and maybe the wrong) things until it's too late. Eliminating the test won't help; throwing away the bathroom scales won't end obesity or stop it becoming a disease.

Another important criticism of medicine is its vertical approach—the relationship between you and your doctor is vertical. You are the subordinate member in that relationship. The doctor is the dominant one. He or she is the alpha baboon, in anthropological terms. And the entire system is calculated to make sure that you understand that, know your place.

So you make an appointment to see a doctor, often weeks from when you really want one (it's easier to get a prime table at the latest trendy Manhattan restaurant). You take a day off from work and show up on time at the office. You work your way through several layers of predoctor encounters, fill out a bunch of forms, and after having done all that, you cool your heels in a waiting room packed with other subordinate human beings in various degrees of obvious distress, for half an hour or more, thumbing absently through old copies of *People* magazine. Finally you are deposited in an eight-by-ten-foot examining room with nauseating green walls, smelling faintly of disinfectant, and in a skimpy gown with an open back that is supposed to be secured by little ties that you can't possibly reach. You deposit your bare glutei on a cold exam table and wait a while longer for the person you made the appointment to see to show up. By then you are humbled, thoroughly aware of your place in this relationship. The doctor breezes in, and after a fifteen-minute blitzkrieg of verbal and physical assaults (practice managers time these encounters), you are told to do or take something, are given a prescription, and Dr. Alpha Baboon is off to his or her next victim. This is a vertical relationship, and it is very clear that you're not the one on top.

This kind of medicine doesn't work very well even for people who are sick. About a third of the prescriptions doctors write are never filled. No more than half of the patients who see a doctor actually do what the doctor thinks he or she told them to do. That is true even for people like Mr. Hensley, who have a disease that has serious consequences if medications aren't taken. He didn't take his insulin and wound up in a coma in a hospital emergency room and shortly thereafter, dead.

Sometimes the problem is communication. Several years ago a young couple presented at a hospital emergency room about 1:00 a.m. on a frigid winter night. By the time they were seen by the resident on duty, they had waited for a couple of hours. The young woman had a fever and unmistakable signs of a kidney infection. She was also very obviously pregnant.

The resident asked, "When are you due?"

The young woman's face went blank.

Her husband answered, "What do you mean?"

"I mean when is she due to deliver the baby?" the resident responded.

"She's not pregnant," he answered. "She can't be. We're using the pill."

Of course the pill is not a hundred percent effective, the resident knew, so he asked, "Did she miss any days taking the pill?"

A broad, proud smile broke across the young man's face and he said, "Oh, sir, I take the pill and I haven't missed a single day. I've always felt that birth control is the man's responsibility."

What a doctor thinks he told a patient to do and what the patient understood can be quite different. Fifteen minutes doesn't allow very much time for explanations. Ruth Parker, a doctor at Emory who studies health literacy, spends most of her professional time at Grady Memorial Hospital, the public institution that serves, among others, the indigent of Fulton and DeKalb counties in Georgia. Her findings are enlightening. The gap between what health-care providers think patients are instructed to do or take and what the patient hears and does is enormous. Dr. Parker has a series of filmed interviews with patients exploring that chasm, and what they reveal is truly amazing (see http://www.acpfoundation.org/hl/hlresources.htm). It is tempting to think that what medical professionals need most is a course in Communication 101.

Failure of communication is one of the problems, but as important as that is, it is not the only reason for the disconnect between prescription and practice. There is a whole catalog of explanations for why people don't do what they are told, even if they and the doctor are on the same page: They can't afford the medicine, they don't think it's important, they forget, the doctor isn't convincing enough, it's too much trouble, they're too busy, etc. And these are people who have a medical condition that needs attention. The current system fails even more miserably to get essentially healthy people to do the things that will make them healthier; most doctors don't spend much time trying. The payoff is so small, why bother?

But sometimes people do change. Young men return from war forever changed. A religious epiphany can cause people to behave differently, as can surviving a cardiac arrest or dealing successfully with a life-threatening cancer—there is a long list of life-changing experiences that cause people to make a U-turn, head in a different direction.

Take Leann Hendrix. In 1998 she won the Miss Arizona beauty contest. Obviously beautiful, she was also an athlete, swimming competitively since she was four. In 2002 she injured her leg while working out. A blood clot formed, a piece of which dislodged, eventually clogging an artery supplying blood to a critical part of her brain. She had a stroke. She couldn't remember a lot of her past. Her longtime boyfriend deserted her. She had to relearn how to walk. But Ms. Hendrix also became an articulate and dedicated champion of stroke victims. She travels around the country talking to support groups. She lobbies Congress. She even appeared on *Larry King Live*. A stroke can be a life-changing event.

Dramatic emotional, social, and physical events can change people. But there is no reason why one must have a stroke, get cancer, or nearly die before being sufficiently motivated to pay attention to one's own or others' health. Some creativity is in order, but we can do some things differently than we are doing them now.

A key component of this new way of doing things is a horizontal partnership between the essentially healthy person and a health-care professional. We call this new breed of health professionals "health partners" to emphasize the fundamental nature of what they do and how they do it. New programs and new kinds of professionals already exist that are attempting to address the issue. There are health-care programs that employ "health coaches" or "health mentors" to help people manage chronic illnesses like diabetes or heart failure. Those programs appear to work. Chronic diseases are better cared for in that setting. The concept extended to healthy people, before they get a chronic illness, has even greater potential. The idea would be to engage healthy people in a partnership with a health-care professional, who would share responsibility for their health, provide information, help navigate the health-care system when necessary, and provide moral support for the tough task of changing lifestyle.

These health partners have five key tasks: engage, educate, empower, promote, and observe. They engage in a mutual effort to educate participants about their health, empower them to take control of environments and behaviors where there are opportunities to become healthier, and promote healthy change and honest observation over the long haul. The mnemonic E³PO is a near homophone of a *Star Wars* character, but these are not aliens, even though their role may be alien to the current health-care system. They are very much attuned to the earthly experiences of real human beings.

Engagement requires more than lip service. Getting real engagement may be the biggest battle in the personal health war. The personal interactions with the heath partner and the physical experience in our center, where partners and participants interact, are designed to get participants' attention, to cause them to care about their health.

Education means giving essentially healthy people more information about their total state of health—mind, body, and spirit—than they will learn in any other program. The health partner explains where the opportunities are: the good, the bad, and the ugly, and also the realistic possibilities.

Empowerment invests participants with the responsibility and power to take control of their own health and well-being. There are ways to improve, most of which are neither impossible nor even that difficult. Most important, these efforts are tailored to where and how an individual lives. The partner helps the participant plot a realistic course.

Promotion is cheerleading in a sense, but also being a voice of reason and objectivity, solidly on the participant's side but not an enabler of bad behaviors. Fundamental to the relationship is persistence—whether or not a participant reaches a goal, the health partner doesn't go away. You can count on it.

Observation addresses the fact that we are terrible observers of ourselves, very bad at seeing ourselves as others see us, to paraphrase Robert Burns. A health partner is a sympathetic but objective observer, helping each participant deal with the reality of who and where he or she is. The partner brings sympathetic, caring, value-neutral objectivity to the relationship.

In our experience at Emory, this horizontal arrangement is likely a major factor in the program's high retention rate—the overwhelming majority of people entering the program do stick with it. Participants have given a variety of reasons for staying with the program, but many say they continue to be attracted to the idea of deciding for themselves what to do and then having help doing it, rather than being told what to do and being berated for failing.

There is no single source for such partners. Those in the Emory program are not doctors, nurses, nurse practitioners, or any other currently recognized health professional. We value people skills more than academic focus, so our health partners come from diverse educational backgrounds, holding bachelor's degrees in biology, education, exercise science, nutrition, psychology, and communication. Some have master's degrees as well. Several have had some experience in health-related people interactions, but all have undergone a four-month intense didactic and practical training that includes indoctrination in the fundamental concepts of Predictive Health, as well as all the measurements taken in the center; training in technical skills necessary for the tests we use; formal training in empathetic, active listening; experience in motivational interviewing and assessment of readiness to change; and training in collaborative decision making and goal setting and goal-directed problem solving. The curriculum contains elements of health coaching, mentoring, and supportive engagement. Each partner-in-training then shadows an experienced one during participant interactions and when deemed ready for action is shadowed by an experienced partner for several of the initial participant encounters. As we have seen, the program retains participants at a high level, so we think it likely that we're onto something here.

To come full circle back to Christensen, for Predictive Health to be truly disruptive, it has to be much less expensive than the system we have now. The health partner is indeed a lot less expensive than doctors, nurses, and the like, and a single partner can follow at least a hundred, maybe many more, essentially healthy people. We will still need physicians and other, more expensive, skilled health professionals, but the activities of a health partner should decrease the demand for their skills substantially. What's more, the economic impact of this system for participants should be more than savings on medical bills, because improved health and well-being will reduce days out of work; improve efficiency while at work; allow people to have longer, productive lives; and generally improve their satisfaction with life.

Professor Bill Rouse and his colleagues in the industrial systems engineering department at Georgia Tech are working on putting numbers to these benefits. Using real information from the Emory Georgia Tech Center for Health Discovery and Well Being®, they're developing detailed economic models that should be enlightening and should enable us to tailor Predictive Health to emphasize those components that have the greatest impact on health and well-being and are most cost effective.

A final indication of the disruptive potential of these partnerships for health care is the possibility that health partners will make themselves obsolete, at least for a number of participants. Although caring for health and well-being is a lifelong commitment, if the partnership works as it should, it may be more of a transition period during which a participant learns to engage, educate, empower, promote, and observe on his or her own. Maybe after a while the need for the partnership will diminish or go away. With time and experience (the time will be highly individual), each of us may graduate to become his or her own health partner.

Ms. Echt did this pretty much on her own; she was engaged in caring for her health. But she was blessed with considerable resources and better opportunities than most people. Even so, we think there is a good chance that a more intimate partnering with a health-focused professional would have spared her some trouble. Speculation about Mr. Hensley is more certain. Given the opportunity to participate in this approach to caring for his health, we are convinced that he would have lived longer and better. It is also likely that over his lifetime a lot of medical care dollars would have gone unspent. And that, for even the most steely-eyed accountant, would be real disruption.

PART IV

The Broader View

The territory of health as an individual and collective human condition includes the humanities (literature, music, dance, art, religion, drama), architecture, sociology, law, business, economics, policy, engineering. The possibility of programs that fully integrate those areas of expertise with biology, public health, and the more applied disciplines of nursing and medicine is the kind of opportunity that should cause imaginative academicians to salivate.

CHAPTER 16

The Tyranny of Paradigm

The hills are shadows, and they flow
From form to form, and nothing stands;
They melt like mist, the solid lands,
Like clouds they shape themselves and go.

———————

Alfred Lord Tennyson, *In Memoriam A.H.H.*

You have brains in your head.
You have feet in your shoes.
You can steer yourself any direction you choose.
You're on your own. And you know what you know.
And you are the one who'll decide where to go. . . .

———————

Dr. Seuss, *Oh, the Places You'll Go!*

ALTHOUGH WE CANNOT predict the timing, we are confident
that health care in the United States is about to undergo some
dramatic changes—and we are not alone in this. We are also fairly
sure that a major part of that change will be a shift in emphasis and
resources toward defining health as a complete and dynamic human

experience rather than a static fact of biology and using that new knowledge to keep people healthy. This will happen because it can. The explosion of discovery in the relevant sciences and technologies is revealing possibilities that stretch our imaginations.

But making Predictive Health a reality is not about the science. Well, it is about the science, but that's going to happen anyway—curiosity and the drive to scratch that intellectual itch are so innately human that discovery will happen, one way or another. Realizing Predictive Health is more about paradigms of the sort that Thomas Kuhn discussed in his seminal book *The Structure of Scientific Revolutions*.

A wag once said that he didn't know what a paradigm was, but he knew that it was always shifting. That's certainly not true in the world of medicine. How biomedicine is done and paid for in America changes direction with all the speed and agility of the *Titanic* in the open sea. Systemic inertia is not unique to medicine and health care, of course. Kuhn, a physicist and philosopher of science, dealt with paradigms and how they change in science, but concepts can ossify in any aspect of life. His observations and conclusions have important ramifications for the shift from disease-oriented medicine to the much more broadly conceived biomedicine that we advocate for Predictive Health.

The big advances in science, Kuhn argues, are not an inevitable result of steady accretions of facts, a product of what he calls "normal science." Such science is slave to accepted notions. It labors to fit experimental observations into the prevailing paradigm. If an observation doesn't fit the paradigm, one assumes that the experiment was a dud; something wasn't controlled just right. That must be true, because the unquestioned assumption is that the paradigm is right. The result was an anomaly. But enough anomalies can trigger a crisis, typically resisted until a new paradigm prevails (a paradigm shift), which lasts until the cycle repeats itself. Copernicus's and Galileo's challenge of the Ptolemaic, Earth-centered cosmology is an archetypal case. The really interesting thing about how paradigms shift is that scientific advance is not a strictly logical, fact-driven result of business as usual—it's an overturning of deeply held cultural beliefs and practices. Major advances are not incremental, but rather a result of episodic, revolutionary change in fundamental assumptions. And that change happens, even in the sciences, as a cultural phenomenon, a consequence of interactions of ideas, data, social pressures, personalities, world conditions, and subjective perceptions of human beings and their universe. Science "as usually done" doesn't drive even change within itself except as a part of a social miasma—culture.

Exploding science and technology will enable change. The omics, information technology, and innovative devices will make it possible to measure, understand, and affect health in new ways, in different places, and with different health professionals than the way we do these things now. Science and technology will make Predictive Health possible. But change will only happen because it must, because it becomes a cultural imperative. And we are already at that point. We simply cannot afford or forever justify spending more and more money on care while becoming less and less healthy. The current younger generation of Americans may be the first to have a shorter life expectancy than their parents as health-care costs continue their skyrocketing trajectory toward bankruptcy. The persisting quandary is whether there will be sufficient social sanity to effect positive systemic change before a health-care Armageddon forces the issue. We see three major potential forces for change—politics, economics, and education—although we doubt that all three will realize that potential. Will they foster change, and will it come via the chaos of revolution or a more ordered process of evolution? We cannot confidently predict.

Political systems are not incapable of effecting major health-related change. The story of Luther Leonidas Terry, son of an Alabama small town doctor, who became President John F. Kennedy's surgeon general in 1961, is proof. At least since the 1950s, evidence had been mounting that cigarette smoking was a significant risk factor for lung cancer, chronic bronchitis, emphysema, and probably cardiovascular disease. A 1962 report from the British Royal College of Physicians made the evidence even clearer, prompting Terry to appoint an advisory committee on the subject, which he chaired. The committee's report, *Smoking and Health: Report of the Committee to the Surgeon General of the United States,* was released on January 11, 1964. Its impact, though not immediate, was profound.

In 1964, cigarette smoking was an American cultural phenomenon. Over half of adult men and almost half of the entire American population smoked. Free sample five-packs of cigarettes were routinely doled out on airplanes. Office workers smoked while working at their desks. Restaurants, theaters, all kinds of public places were smoker friendly. College classrooms, even medical school lecture rooms, were often thick with cigarette smoke, with medical professors smoking even while delivering lectures! And "Big Tobacco" was, of course, big business. Taking that on took some courage. But Luther Terry, a Red Level, Alabama, boy made good, took on Big Tobacco, with major consequences.

The battle between human health and cigarette smoke rages on, but less in America than elsewhere, and with a different set of rules since the Terry report. According to the CDC, half as many Americans smoked in 2010 as did in 1964. Smoking in public places is mostly illegal. Advertising is strictly limited, and conspicuous health warnings are required on cigarette packages. Tobacco companies have lost major health-related lawsuits, costing them billions. Presently in the United States of America, smoking is not generally socially acceptable behavior. The paradigm has shifted.

We have less confidence, however, that modern politics can effect such lasting and important positive change in health care as a whole. Health-care reform has been in the political circus's center ring in recent years, with too much misinformation, too many private interests, and too little concern for the public good. The volume of the self-serving "misinfomercials" has been far too high. According to the Pew Research Center for People and the Press, in the last six months of 2009, nearly half the news stories about health-care reform were about politics, and only 9 percent dealt with substantive issues. Not surprisingly, the American public has gotten lost in the noise; the Pew survey found that 69 percent of Americans didn't understand the debate in December 2009. The issues are complex, the implications enormous, and the risk of unintended consequences real. The solution is likely to be disruptive, and disruption tends to attract vocal controversy and isn't often a big vote-getter. The political process is also very adept at denying impending cataclysm for as long as possible—consider climate change, or even the prolonged battle over cigarettes, which lasted well into the 1990s. The political process just doesn't lend itself to dramatic change until the threat of disaster looms undeniably large.

Even when there is a will to do something—such as with health care in 2009—what ultimately gets done might bear little resemblance to the initial intent, as deals cut to mollify entrenched interests and power brokers in and out of Congress macerate even the noblest of goals in the political sausage grinder. We are not optimistic about a political solution, at least not within our lifetimes.

Some political intransigence is due to pressures from corporations and their lobbyists—this was obviously the case during the battle over smoking, and many segments of the health-care industry are satisfied with where they are and are willing to fight tooth and nail to stay there—but it is possible that emerging economic imperatives can drive change as effectively as old imperatives might hinder it. Certainly it is true that what gets paid for is what will be done, so if private insurance companies, health systems, and employers decide to move toward a focus on health, they can make it happen. There has been some promising movement in that direction.

Several large hospitals and health-care systems, including Northwestern Memorial Hospital in Chicago, the Mayo Clinic, Kaiser Permanente, Geisinger Health System, Vanderbilt University Medical Center, and Ascension Health, have developed dedicated innovation centers, modeled after corporate entities that test new production methods, work processes, physical spaces, and new approaches to customer service. Lyle Berkowitz, founder of Northwestern Memorial's Szollosi Healthcare Innovation Program, describes the rationale bluntly: It is better to "make changes now rather than wait until the system collapses." Fear is a potent motivator.

By and large these programs are still focused on innovation in delivery of disease care, although there is at least one exception. Kaiser Permanente has developed a cadre of programs focused on both well-being and physical health. Kaiser Permanente Thrive is a particularly attractive one. The program emphasizes health as an integrated phenomenon of mind, body, and spirit; its advertising tag line, "we want you to thrive," contrasts with the more common and negative disease prevention approach. Kaiser Permanente is not primarily a benevolent society, and the medical groups involved are for-profit entities; if they aren't driven by a profit motive, then they aren't doing their fiduciary duty. So we suppose that the decision makers at KP believe that this emphasis on health and well-being will pay off. We hope it does.

Employers, bedeviled by health-care costs, are also recognizing that wellness programs for their workers are a good investment. An article in the December 2010 *Harvard Business Review* titled, "What's the Hard Return on Employee Wellness Programs?" reviews some of those experiences. The leaders of Johnson and Johnson, for example, estimate that their employee wellness programs saved the company $250 million over the previous decade, with each dollar invested between 2002 and 2008 returning $2.71. Another study of a random sample of 185 workers and their spouses by Richard Milani and Carl Lavie produced even more dramatic results. The subjects were essentially healthy working people who were enrolled in a wellness program during the study. By the end of a six-month program, each person's medical claim costs had decreased by almost $1,500 from the previous year. The return on each dollar invested was a whopping $6.00.

Employers also save money because healthy workers are better workers. MD Anderson Cancer Center's employee health and well-being department programs decreased their employees' lost work time by 80 percent, saving $1.5 million in paid sick leave. Workers also stick with companies with highly effective wellness programs, driving down the cost of turnover.

Maybe there is reason to feel encouraged about these stirrings of the sleeping economic giant. Many disruptive advances in American society have been driven by economic motives, so why not in health care?

There is one powerful reason why not. Realizing the full potential of Predictive Health will take more than KP Thrive and the MD Anderson employee health and well-being department. Bringing the best that the humanities, the sciences, and technology have to contribute to human health to the marketplace in American society will require the knowledge and practice of a universe of disciplines—law, business, human behavior, religion, sociology, anthropology, health policy, public health—virtually every area of inquiry relevant to the human experience. And the real challenge is that this catalog of experts will have to learn to converse with each other and with basic and clinical scientists, all of whom speak different languages and think in different ways. Economics can't make that happen, but perhaps universities can.

We admit to a bias here; our entire professional lives have been spent in the service of universities. But our belief in the potential of universities to effect change is not just brash parochialism. Universities have much to bring to the table, not just because of the experts who live, work, and play there, but because they thrive on discovery and innovation. They are less constrained by convention and the pressure for urgent payoffs than the private sector is. At their best, universities foster—and their faculties relish—challenging accepted dogma. Whereas businesses may fear disruption because it threatens their modus operandi, universities are less vulnerable to disruptive innovation and so are freer to assail the unassailable than institutions that depend for their survival on more immediate consequences of what they do. What's more, universities are where the rising generations are educated, attitudes are formed, passions nurtured, causes seized, knowledge acquired, and skills developed.

There is at least one major problem, however. Redesigning health care—which may be the single greatest opportunity for universities to help humanity in this century, perhaps this millennium—cannot be done by "multiversities," with diverse experts thwarted at common tasks like the builders of the tower of Babel. Institutions must learn to integrate diverse pursuits, to focus intellectual lights from all directions on a common challenge, to behave in a manner worthy of their name. That would be another major paradigm shift, as academic territories are often jealously guarded, but universities and even medical education have proven capable of major change before.

At the turn of the twentieth century there were over 150 medical schools in America. There were no rules, standards, or required accreditation. Many were proprietary schools, run for profit by an entrepreneurial doctor or two whose own training was as spotty as the education they were selling. At the same time, there was a competing paradigm. A handful of university-associated medical schools had more rigorous admission standards and curricula that included the basic and clinical sciences and obligatory laboratory and dissection experiences, as well as strict standards for graduating. The result was two different kinds of doctors and two different kinds of medical practice.

Most people didn't seem to mind. If the doctor was amiable and available and seemed to know what he or she was doing, that was enough. Given how little even the best-educated physicians had to work with, maybe patients weren't missing that much if their doctor was a quack.

But change came. It started when the American Medical Association's Council on Medical Education laid out a set of criteria for the training of doctors and asked the Carnegie Foundation for the Advancement of Teaching to do a survey of the current state of affairs. The survey was led by an esteemed educator named Abraham Flexner, who went at the job with a vengeance. He visited every one of the existing schools, turning on them the hard eye of the progressive educator that he was, and he pulled no punches in his evaluations. Of Chicago's fourteen medical schools he wrote that they were, "a disgrace to the State whose laws permit its existence . . . indescribably foul . . . the plague spot of the nation." His report—published in 1910 as Carnegie Foundation Bulletin no. 4, but usually known as the "Flexner Report"—is the document that changed the paradigm. It recommended admission requirements that were at that time met by only 16 of the existing 155 medical schools in the United States and Canada, stipulated a four-year medical curriculum containing the CME recommendations, and stated that all proprietary schools should either close or be subsumed into existing universities. By 1935 the number of medical schools was down to 66, almost all university affiliated. State medical boards adopted the report's standards and started enforcing them. The new paradigm was universally accepted, and the nature of medical education and consequently practice was changed into what is essentially the current model.

There are of course many other examples of changing paradigms, although most are not very encouraging. In chapter 11 we mention Ignatz Semmelweis, driven to distraction by the resistance of his profession to his revolutionary concept of the cause and demonstrated prevention for lethal childbed fever. Barry Marshall had to take on a billion-dollar industry and an entrenched concept in order to realize the consequences of his discovery that gastric ulcers are infectious. Medicine was slow to appreciate the health hazards of radiation and asbestos exposure. The list is long.

Perhaps we belabor the point that major change—and Predictive Health would be a major change—does not come quickly or easily. Even in science, change is a complex product of facts, attitudes, private interests, public opinion, political trade winds, and much else. But our admission of potential problems is not an admission of defeat. Indeed, there are already some university programs that aim to integrate expertise to address health in that fog of resonating signals where biology, behavior, and environment overlap. To illustrate this we mention two programs from very different parts of the world. Although we cannot vouch for how well either of the programs is meeting its stated goals, we are impressed by the territory they have staked out for themselves.

Researchers in the Human Health and Wellbeing Domain of the Institute of Health and Biomedical Innovation at Queensland University of Technology in Brisbane, Australia, are focused on "developing and evaluating interventions that will prevent disease, promote health and well being and improve care." A cadre of academicians concentrates on social and environmental issues, healthy aging, health in children and adolescents, and mental health and well-being. In addition to its academic programs, the institute works with industry to implement health-focused care programs for people of all ages. Its members serve as personal health consultants to aid small businesses in developing evidence-based health management plans for their employees. These goals are laudable, and the approaches appear to be unconstrained by disciplinary boundaries; biology, environment, and behavior are viewed as integrated definers of health. And the participants connect to the community to get things done. We don't know how well it works, but the concept seems spot on.

The University of Pittsburgh's Center for Research on Health Care partners with that institution's Clinical and Translational Science Institute, the Center for Health Equity Research and Promotion, and the RAND–University of Pittsburgh Health Institute as a sort of consortium of people and approaches to innovation in health care. They have created a collaborative center for developing ideas into feasible projects. They nurture interdisciplinary investigative teams and aim to increase communication and collaboration among the university's component departments and schools. This seems like a positive direction. No doubt they face the challenges typical of virtually all American university administrative structures. But we applaud the attempt.

There are numerous other examples; we chose these two at random as illustrations. The support of clinical and translational science centers by the National Institutes of Health at several American universities is a focused attempt to move discovery from the laboratory to benefit people; those centers are required to be interdisciplinary. But how interdisciplinary? There seems to be an as-yet-unoccupied space for discovery and innovation that would expand the concept of interdisciplinarity. The territory of health as an individual and collective human condition includes the humanities (literature, music, dance, art, religion, drama), architecture, sociology, law, business, economics, policy, and engineering. The possibility of programs fully integrating those areas of expertise with biology, public health, and the more applied disciplines of nursing and medicine is the kind of opportunity that should cause imaginative academicians to salivate.

Some seeds are being sown, but it may be too late for these kinds of efforts to do much for people of our generation. Existing organizations may not be enough. To change the course of health care, we have to reach the coming generations—graduate students and undergraduates, certainly, but even that may be too late a start if we really expect to change culture. Still, reorienting much of health-related education at all levels could pave the way for the coming waves of graduates to see the challenges with new eyes and approach solutions with creativity unrestrained by history and unintimidated by the prevailing paradigm.

Institutions of higher learning are beginning to get the message. Graduate programs are emerging in areas such as social sciences and health research, politics and sociology, mind-body medicine, nursing business and health systems, and health-care innovation. There are joint degree programs among professional schools (medicine, business, engineering, law, nursing, public health). A program known as Undergraduate Medical Education for the 21st Century, sponsored by the federal Health Resources and Services Administration, is meant to introduce innovative educational experiences for doctors in training. The rationale is that current medical education poorly prepares graduates for practicing medicine in the settings where they will spend their professional lives. The program is funded in eighteen medical schools, which work with fifty external organizations (a variety of health entities) to include different experiences for medical students, mostly focused on disease care rather than health care.

A graduate program recently created by the Burroughs Wellcome Foundation deserves special mention. That foundation has funded three doctorate level programs, which were selected from many more applications, with the explicit requirement that they bridge laboratory and population sciences. The program, housed in the Laney Graduate School at Emory (we call it Molecules to Mankind—M2M), engages faculty from medicine, public health, anthropology, and biology. Each student must have a particular interest in learning multiple disciplines and conducting research in both a laboratory and a population science; one of the tracks is in Predictive Health, exploiting the transinstitutional strategic theme. These are new programs (at Emory only the second group of students is being chosen), but the initial experience has excited faculty and students. The demand is already outstripping the available slots. A parallel undergraduate curriculum—consistently oversubscribed—draws lecturers from medicine, public health, sociology, philosophy, ethics, anthropology, engineering, genetics, psychiatry/psychology, and elsewhere (partnerships with Georgia Tech and the nearby CDC create an incredibly rich source of faculty). We are encouraged to think that these kinds of novel approaches to health-related education will make a difference. As in many areas, we may have to trust the coming generations to clean up the mess we have made of health care. The least we can do is everything we can think of to equip them for the task.

The biomedical sciences juggernaut will continue to give us new understandings of human biology and increasingly more sophisticated tools for measuring vital processes. The possibilities will multiply well beyond anything we can imagine now. But our collective ability to realize the enormous benefit that science promises has a long way to go. Political solutions, if they occur at all, will not come quickly enough to avoid some serious consequences of the path we are on. Maybe capitalism will drive transformative change in this area, as it has done in others. There are suggestive rumblings afoot. But the profit motive tends more toward incremental than disruptive innovation. The phenomenal opportunity for integrating a broad swath of disciplines to address the many and complex facets of the problem, to imagine and create transformation, is the elephant that stalks the halls of academe, largely unnoticed. We may have to patch things together for a while, temporize, until the coming generations view the opportunity with new eyes and unencumbered brains and fix the problem for us. The good news is that the generations incubating in our schools, colleges, and universities are a phenomenally gifted, creative, and caring group. They just may be up to the task.

CHAPTER 17

Healthy People—
Healthy Planet

H UMAN HEALTH CANNOT be defined narrowly. We have
made that point by emphasizing health as existing in the space
where biology, environment, and behavior overlap, but we may have
underplayed the role of environment. The bioworld is intercon-
nected and interdependent enough that human health must be defined in a very large context, well beyond the boundaries of our
homes and jobs. For example, if you have asthma only when exposed
to polluted air (the rest of the time you breathe perfectly fine), is
your asthma your disease, or a disease of the atmospheric conditions,
social inclinations, political decisions, manufacturing processes, and
polluting devices that determine what your airways are exposed to?
After all, if whatever pollutes your particular microatmosphere—ni-
trous oxides or whatever—is not what your lungs were made to
breathe, then it seems clear that the disease they provoke is not just
"yours."

Asthma is not the only human affliction that could be viewed as
a disease of ecology; there are many others. Dump billions of cubic
feet of noxious gases into the air, and at least portions of the ill effects will be pretty easily predicted, regardless of individual differences in genomes, proteomes, and metabolomes. The same goes for

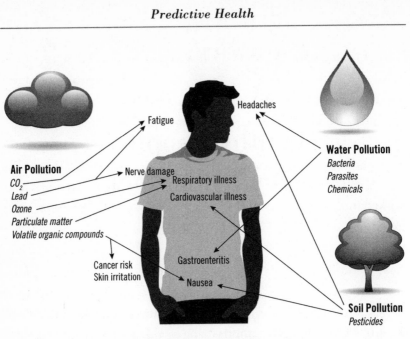

Air Pollution
CO$_2$
Lead
Ozone
Particulate matter
Volatile organic compounds

Fatigue

Headaches

Nerve damage
Respiratory illness
Cardiovascular illness

Cancer risk
Skin irritation

Gastroenteritis

Nausea

Water Pollution
Bacteria
Parasites
Chemicals

Soil Pollution
Pesticides

Health Effects of Pollution

polluting water and food, dumping toxic wastes in places where they leach into things that humans eat and drink. Poison is poison, and the consequences for human health are not going to be good. We can predict that with certainty.

But why would an intelligent human being let himself or herself be exposed to that stuff? After all, there are warning signs—trouble breathing, skin rash, burning eyes, stomach trouble. The above figure illustrates some of these consequences. All other things being equal, those symptoms should motivate us to steer clear of the offending situation. But all other things aren't equal. If there are diseases of personal choice, maybe there are also *diseases of personal necessity*.

In the mid- to late twentieth century, the largest integrated steel plant in the world sprawled across a peninsula separating the Patapsco and Back Rivers on an outer edge of Baltimore, Maryland. More than thirty thousand people worked there. The Bethlehem Steel

Corporation owned the mill and almost everything else in Sparrow's Point. Work in the mill was dirty, hot, and dangerous, but it attracted workers like a magnet because it paid well. For a young man with just a high school education, it paid better than just about anything else he could do in Baltimore. A job at the mill was a ticket to the American dream—your own home, a nice car. And the benefits were good. So it is not surprising that Carleton Hensley, who worked in that mill, stayed there even though his job, like most others in the mill, was dirty, hot, and dangerous. He was a welder, and welders also spent their daily (or nightly; the mill ran three shifts most of the time) eight hours breathing fumes: zinc fumes, tungsten fumes, and carbon monoxide. An acute allergic reaction, called metal fume fever, is common among welders. A daily bout of drinking after work was routine—part of the job, really. When the mill was at its peak, the Sea Horse Inn in neighboring Dundalk, where a lot of workers lived, went through seventy barrels of beer (more than two thousand gallons) a week. It's likely that Mr. Hensley and a cadre of coworkers had a favorite bar where they spent a few hours most every day anesthetizing away the pains and troubles of the job. Drinking might have seemed the best way to deal with the situation; he had mouths to feed, a family to provide for, so he was unlikely to quit. The mill paid too well. Unfortunately, the drinking, the stress, and the stuff he breathed probably contributed to his premature illness and death. But he had to make a living. So perhaps the distinction between diseases of choice and diseases of necessity doesn't make too much sense here. As Upton Sinclair had it, "It is difficult to get a man to understand something when his salary depends on his not understanding."

We call other diseases caused by environmental pollution that one can't easily avoid *diseases of circumstance.* You could choose not to live in a city, but if you do live in a large city, chances are you are exposed to potential toxins by just being there—it wasn't just the workers in the 1960s steel mill who suffered ill effects. History is full of dramatic examples of what a disease of circumstance looks like. Some at least served a useful purpose by calling attention to the dangers and triggering social action.

It is possible that Donora, Pennsylvania, a sleepy mill town a few miles southeast of Pittsburgh, would have merited a footnote in baseball history (Cardinal great Stan Musial was born there, as were Ken Griffey senior and junior), but it's virtually certain that the town would not have made it into the *New Yorker* magazine or Berton Roueche's *Eleven Blue Men* (the book that made epidemiology sexy) except for the events of October 27–31, 1948. From October 27, when the smog first rolled down the Monongahela River, until the blessed rain came on October 31, a toxic pall, trapped under the weight of an unusual temperature inversion, bathed the town's fourteen thousand residents in a dense yellow acrid effluvium spewing from the Donora Zinc Works and its American Steel and Wire Plant. Twenty Donora residents died, and thousands were made ill; almost a thousand animals also died. Another fifty people died later (including Lukasz Musial, Stan's father) as a direct result of the smog, and hundreds more suffered lung and heart problems for the rest of their shortened lives. The Donora smog was a wake-up call. An unhealthy planet Earth is an unhealthy habitat for humans and other animals! Pollution can kill and maim! The social passions that the incident stirred are credited with starting the clean air movement in the United States. And although it was a long time coming, the Clean Air Act of 1970 probably had its roots in Donora.

By 1952 Londoners were used to fog, even dense fog, *peasoupers*, saturated with soot from the coal fires most homes used for heating. So it wasn't immediately obvious that that year was any different, although in retrospect, Londoners called it the Great Smog of '52 or Big Smoke. It rolled in on Friday, December 5, and didn't leave until a fresh wind blew it off down the Thames on Tuesday, December 9. And it killed. When the bodies were counted over that week and for several weeks thereafter, death rates were discovered to be several times normal, with the smog having probably killed more than twelve thousand people and sickened thousands more. Poisoned environments poison the people who inhabit them. A galvanized British government moved to enact legislation. The Clean Air Act of 1956 authorized establishment of smokeless zones and provided grants for converting home heating from coal to gas, oil, or electricity.

Many of the deaths in Donora in 1948 and London in 1952 were from heart and lung ailments. Some victims already had breathing or circulation problems, and the smog just made them worse, but many others did not. The smog alone was toxic enough to their hearts and lungs to make them sick or die. But an unhealthy planet may not just injure hearts and lungs. There may be less dramatic but more fundamental effects on human health.

Two epidemiologists, J. C. Chen and J. Schwartz, knew that breathing polluted air had been shown to cause at least biochemical evidence of both inflammation and oxidant stress, which underlie most chronic illnesses. And they knew that people with metabolic syndrome—the condition in which obesity, high blood pressure, diabetes, and high blood lipids exist together—may also react more vigorously to polluted air than other people breathing the same air. Chen and Schwartz investigated the relationships among inflammation, metabolic syndrome, and pollution. They retrieved metabolic syndrome and inflammation related data from the National Health and Nutrition Examination Survey and air quality data (they used the concentration of very small particles as their quality metric) from the U.S. Environmental Protection Agency Aerometric Information Retrieval System. They then superimposed the two sets of data. When they looked at white blood cell count as a

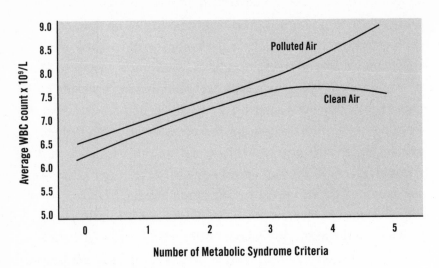

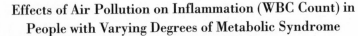

**Effects of Air Pollution on Inflammation (WBC Count) in
People with Varying Degrees of Metabolic Syndrome**

Source: Redrawn from data in J. C. Chen and J. Schwartz, "Metabolic Syndrome
and Inflammatory Responses to Long-term Particulate Air Pollutants,"
Environmental Health Perspectives 116 (2008): 612–617.

measure of inflammation, they found that people breathing polluted air had on average more inflammation whether or not they
had any evidence of metabolic syndrome. And when they separated people into groups based on how many of the five criteria
for metabolic syndrome they met, the members of each group
showed more inflammation the more polluted air they breathed;
what's more, the effect was more dramatic the worse the metabolic
syndrome (see the figure above). Breathing unhealthy air is bad for
people whether they are basically healthy or not, but the effect is
even worse if they are not that healthy to begin with. Maybe there
is a vicious cycle where an unhealthy planet makes unhealthy people and then keeps adding insult to injury.

So we can see how an unhealthy planet makes people unhealthy
and, by inference, how a healthy earth environment would promote

health. Could this work in the opposite direction? Will people who are healthy (and by that we mean in the integrated Predictive Health sense) make the planet healthier?

Maybe. Some research has attempted to correlate characteristics of individual people who behave as though they are concerned about the fate of the planet—they buy locally grown foods, choose green cleaning products, are conscious of energy use, select high gas-mileage cars, etc.—with other facts about them or their behaviors. At least some of the green behaviors correlate with age, income, and educational level; no big surprises there. Interestingly, there does seem to be a relationship between a person's feeling of control over external events and both concern about the environment and behaviors reflecting that concern. This is interesting because a number of public health advocates think that a person's sense of control over external events is an important variable in determining general health and that this may account for some socioeconomic health disparities.

So individual behaviors may help to make our planet healthier, and it may be that, as Al Gore admonishes in *An Inconvenient Truth*, "By educating ourselves and others, by doing our part to minimize our use and waste of resources, by becoming more politically active and demanding change . . . each of us can make a difference." But the way our society works, it's not so easy for a lot of people. For people like Mr. Hensley, making a living is the top priority; more distant and grander concerns have to take a back seat. It seems to us that a large share of the responsibility for the health of our planet requires collective concern and action. Governments have the legislative stick to drive social changes that consider our collective health and that of the planet, but as has become all too clear in recent years, wielding that stick takes more dedication and courage than a collection of legislators can often muster. And a lot of fingers, at least since the Industrial Revolution, have been pointed in the direction of corporations.

Some recent actions encourage us to believe that really healthy people, even when grouped into organizations hell-bent on making money, will not be party forever to a rampant fouling of the human nest. It seems that enlightened self-interest, even disregarding the larger human concern about the consequences for the earth and its occupants, should be enough. Could it be that the corporate world, more facile and pragmatic than is often true of government, will emerge to lead the charge toward realizing the natural synergy of humans and nature?

The public battle of Coke with Pepsi over who has the most petroleum-free bottles is an example. Those corporations must believe a lot of people care about that; good for the market. Indeed, Jeffrey Immelt, the chairman of General Electric, put it quite succinctly: "We think green means green." And there is reason to believe that the people who run those mega-businesses care about their planet as well.

The U.S. economy is no longer so dependent on toxin-belching steel plants, and both corporations and universities are paying much more attention to how green they are. Corporate boards are paying close attention to their companies' green initiatives, and universities are insisting on Leed certification for new buildings. We, the collective we, are paying more attention to how what we do affects our planet; we are making real progress.

Theodor Roszak's *The Voice of the Earth* outlines a new field he calls ecopsychology. He writes, "We need a new discipline that sees the needs of the planet and the needs of the person as a continuum and that can help us reconnect with the truth that lies in our communion with the rest of creation." Whether or not you buy the creation thing or the need for yet another discipline, something there is worth pondering. Maller and colleagues refer a little more pragmatically to "contact with nature as an upstream health promotion intervention for populations." They point out that humans have positive biological reactions to animals, plants, and wilderness; natural environments foster recovery from mental fatigue; people seek natural places for solace and rest and recreation; and there are nature-based therapies (horticultural, animal-related) that work. The state of Oregon launched a public health program called Healthy Places, Healthy People in 2008. The rationale wasn't primarily to give Oregonians more recreational opportunities for the sake of recreation; the reason for this multipronged approach to promoting healthy lifestyles was that "together, heart disease, stroke, cancers, diabetes and chronic lower respiratory diseases account for more than three of five deaths in Oregon." The reasoning was that getting people to behave differently and in healthy environments would make for healthier, happier citizens and would decrease health-related costs.

The obligatory resonance among biology, behavior, and environment is the territory of Predictive Health. And any argument about how to prioritize those factors is specious; they cannot be separated from each other. Methods may differ, interventions may vary, but both information and action in any area must be viewed from the middle of the Venn diagram in chapter 3. A blood pressure pill does not affect blood pressure in isolation. It will have little effect if it is combined with a load of salt or an angry relationship or a scary route home. The effect will vary in the context of behavior and environment. On the other hand, take the person with identical blood pressure in a loving relationship, convince her to eat less salt, and help her find a private, quiet place overlooking a green valley where she can go in the afternoon to relax and wind down, and she may not need a pill at all.

So health is an interaction of humans and their planet. The arrow points both ways. The synergy can be influenced by individuals, but there are necessities and circumstances that aren't so easy to change, as well as choices deliberately made. Full realization of the potential of Predictive Health will require collective action. Our history has some dark spots, but we have learned from those and can learn even more. Governments move slowly, if at all, until forced by cataclysms like the Donora smog or the London Big Smoke. The more subtle— but in the long run probably more serious—health effects of environmental pollution are harder to get legislators excited about. Corporations are starting to catch on, however, and there are hints that they could lead the charge. Saving the planet is probably the greatest opportunity for doing good that corporations will have in this century. And they could do well by doing it . . . green is green.

Maybe if we can help a majority of individual people reach exemplary health, there will be a collective effect on how we interact with each other and our planet. There must be connections among the health of individuals, populations, and the globe.

CHAPTER 18

Toward a Square
Wave Life

S O W H E R E D O we go from here? With corporations, universities, better science, political protest? What moves us away from disease to Predictive Health? To be blunt, the answer is you—how you think about your health has to change. No government health-care bill, insurance package, or cleverly marketed health plan will do it. There can (and should) be support systems, but you will have to decide whether each day you spend as a living and breathing, earthbound creature is a day spent dying or living. Are you plodding day by day downward through a life of steady decay toward inevitable oblivion (or whatever you believe awaits you), each day a step nearer an ignominious end? Or do you choose to spend every day allotted to you as full of the joy and exuberance of life as possible, confining the prequel to that inevitable outcome to a brief period when your time is up? We call the latter choice the square wave life (see the illustration on the next page)—living as healthy as we can be for as long as possible—a choice that seems to us the preferable one. And it is a choice!

In the United States we have evolved a perception of health care as something that is done to sick people by doctors, nurses, and other health professionals. That construct will not make most people healthier. Waiting until people are sick is too late. Waiting for a

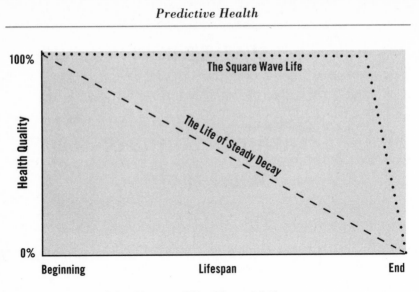

The Shape of Health and Lifespan

stroke to treat high blood pressure is not rational. Even waiting for high blood pressure is missing the real opportunity. And health care should not be something that is delivered to people like Chinese takeout or a Domino's pizza. If we are to lead a square wave life, we will have to be engaged as active participants in the process. Health care should be a mutual effort of knowledgeable, appropriately trained professionals and people who care about themselves. It's about motivation, not compliance. Transforming health care will mean changing the focus by 180 degrees, from the health professional to you, the healthy person.

The transformation must include a change in who the center of attention is and also a change in where health care happens. As long as I have to go to a special place to get all of my health care, I will fail to integrate caring for my health into the way I live. And until I do that, I will not be as healthy as I can be. There is already a trend in disease care away from the traditional hospital. For every thousand Americans, 1,132 nights were spent in a hospital in 1982, down to 607 a decade later. Joe Flower argues in the *Encyclopedia of the Fu-*

ture that the number will be down to 70 or 80 in another decade. That's not enough for Predictive Health, of course; we need health care to move not just away from hospitals but also away from clinics and other medical facilities. In part we expect a migration to workplaces, where we spend much of our time working for people who have a vested interest in our being healthy, thanks to the cost of sick leave, lost productivity, and expensive insurance.

We also spend a lot of time at home. Driven by a shortage of primary care physicians and an increasing prevalence of chronic disease, there is a lot of developing conversation (and some action) around the concept of the medical home. The idea is to make both preventive and curative care accessible and seamless by integrating a broad range of services and involving a spectrum of health professionals. Although this is a concept rather than a physical place, it includes care that happens where a person lives. We would prefer the term to be health home instead of medical home, given our conviction that the real transformation of care is to put health rather than disease in the crosshairs. It also seems to us that every home should be a health home and that realizing the ultimate goal of Predictive Health (keeping people as healthy as they can be for as long as possible—the square wave life) will actually require that. How we live, where we live is the real opportunity for affecting our health. Recall that health is a human condition, an integral part of our everyday experiences, not a simple biological fact. It is a way of living. We don't buy it at the doctor's office.

We also need to transform how we approach tending to our health. We are way too casual about that. Evidence-based health and health-based evidence must link arms with evidence-based medicine and medical practice–based evidence to form the bedrock foundation of health care, the fundamental concept. Science has served us well in many areas, and we should take full advantage of its power to understand health at its most basic level and to find out what works, what doesn't work, and what harms. Science and technology will continue to develop and present new opportunities. The ever-expanding group of omics, nanotechnology, molecular imaging, and unimaginably nimble and capacious bioinformatics will continue to open new doors. We can use those advances to satisfy our wonder about why humans don't get sick more often than they do. Why didn't the epidemics of black plague in Venice in past centuries kill everybody? Why are some people completely resistant to the ravages of the AIDS virus? Why is Jimmy Carter not only alive but apparently well and with a fully functioning brain at past eighty, when legions of his contemporaries waste away in chronic care facilities, unaware of who and where they are? How did Ms. Echt's biology, environment, and behaviors conspire to save her from cancer and a stroke and keep her alive and bright for over a century? We have a better chance to answer questions like these than ever before. And the answers could redefine health-care transformation, presenting possibilities that we can't yet imagine.

Our field of view must also expand. We must see the whole picture, or as much of it as we can, and see ourselves and those for whom we care in that context. We are not independent organisms. We share our space (and most of our biology) with billions of our fellow humans, and we will keep or lose our health in that setting. This focus on health is certainly a personal matter, but not exclusively so. Some things that are vital to our health are necessarily collective concerns. Public health and personal health are integral to each other. They are part of the same spectrum.

Our visual field needs to include health-related practices of all kinds. The vision should be unimpeded by cultural boundaries, academic disciplines, or educational or personal bias. Transformed health care should be integrative in the broadest way that careful observation, sound science, and good judgment permit. Central to our concept of health care should be the realization that we live in that cloud of signals resonating among biology, environment, and behavior.

We will need to transform what and how we teach the coming generations of health professionals. There are real challenges here that we are not meeting very well now. As health care moves ever farther "upstream," away from disease and toward health, we will face new challenges and new opportunities. That health professionals should be trained for what they do and do what they are trained for doesn't seem like a difficult concept, but we, the collective we who are doing the educating, haven't mastered that idea in practice. Presently much health care involves doctors with sophisticated (and expensive) training doing things for which they are overqualified and that they probably do less well than professionals with more focused training could do. We need to look carefully at what kinds of health professionals can best do the jobs in a transformed system and align education with the realities. Cost of care will drive education in that direction, but there is every reason to think that quality of care could also benefit.

But how do we attract the brightest of our youth to a medical profession devoid of emergency room heroics? How do we compete with the glamorized television version of medicine? The whole perception of the profession will have to change. Could it be that we will attract a generation of people who enter the health professions because they care about the health of their fellow persons and feel rewarded by helping people to stay healthy? There will always be a need for ER docs in their soiled scrubs, stethoscopes slung rakishly about their necks. But in a transformed, Predictive Health model of health and healing, we won't need so many of them. And there will be other opportunities for equally rewarding, if less glamorous, careers.

Much of the discussion about health care in America centers on how to create an affordable structure for making disease care, currently available only to the well to do or the well-insured, available to more of our citizens. A lot of the effort is aimed at trying to conceive an approach (including an economic model) that would serve the entire country well, a metaphorical health-care Holy Grail.

But we are a large and diverse country with a very diverse populace, whose health opportunities and risks vary enormously. Is it likely that a single model will work everywhere? There is the same problem in comparing American health-care costs and effectiveness with those of other countries. We really cannot even compare different areas and populations in our own country, much less other countries with different biological, environmental, and social and cultural determinants of behaviors. There is just too much dissimilarity. Patrons of the Cleveland and Mayo clinics are only typical of the patrons of those clinics. They are not at all like the patrons of Grady Memorial Hospital in Atlanta or of the East Harlem Metropolitan Hospital in New York.

We need to transform our approach to health-care policy as well as our approach to practice. More attention must be paid to the numerous microclimates (economic as well as social, ethnic, cultural, and physical) and micropopulations as critical factors in what is possible and what is likely to make those people in those places healthier. The "what" is likely to differ enormously, and so is the "how." Having decided the what (and surely we need to know what needs to be done before designing a way to do it), then a person- and place-specific way to get the job done, the how, can be addressed. But there is not likely to be a single solution to problems that are so very different.

The really big transformation in health and healing is the shift from disease to health, defining health as a complete human experience and perceiving human life at its best as a square wave, health as good as it can be for as long as possible, dying given only the amount of time that's necessary, and accepting death as a natural part of life. That shift in the basic paradigm would drive a lot of change.

EPILOGUE

Life Is a Fatal Condition

A good death does honor to a whole life.

Petrarch, *To Laura in Death*, canzone 16

IF YOU ARE A LIVING human being, sooner or later you will die. If you do not die young, you will age (although we age at different rates) and eventually succumb to something. Even if you escape the big killers—cancer, heart disease, diabetes—you will still die of what we are fond of calling "natural causes." Death is a natural phenomenon that is integral to life. Although science and technology have the potential to dramatically alter the pace and nature of life processes, they will not change the final outcome.

Until you read it, the irony of the title of British writer Julian Barnes's marvelous book on death, *Nothing to Be Frightened Of*, is not obvious (although his facial expression in the picture on the cover is a clue). He spends the 243 pages exploring mortality, his and that of a host of his literary and other acquaintances, with characteristic wit and insight. His perspective is both horizontal (historical) and vertical (his own angst at the prospect). He writes, "I understand (I think) that life depends on death. That we cannot have a planet in the first place without previous deaths of collapsing stars; further, that in order for complex organisms like you and me to inhabit this planet, for there to be self-conscious and self-replacing life, an enormous sequence of evolutionary mutations has had to be tried out and discarded. I can see this, and when I ask, 'Why is death happening to me?' I can applaud theologian John Bowker's crisp reply: 'Because the universe is happening to you.'" We know this, of course. Even if you believe in eternal life, you believe it is something that happens elsewhere, not on the planet and in the physical body where you currently live. We know full well that our conscious experience and that of everyone else with whom we share earthly life is limited in both scope and time. But knowing that death is inevitable as a phenomenon of our species does not mean that we are able to accept the inevitability of the personal experience with equanimity.

One might think that those of us in the medical profession, so familiar with death secondhand (we stand helplessly by and watch people die all the time), would be inured to the experience. But that's not true. In fact, if the goal of a good death is acceptance (having successfully navigated Elisabeth Kubler-Ross's preceding emotional stages of denial, anger, bargaining, and depression), then doctors are worse at it than most. Julian Barnes quotes Sherwin Nuland (a surgeon and author of *How We Die*) as saying, "of all the professions, medicine is the one most likely to attract people with high personal anxieties about dying." Or maybe it comes with the territory. We are forever haunted by that venerable ethos that death is the enemy we are trying to defeat, that the death of someone we are caring for is a personal and professional failure. It is a very short distance from there to denying our own mortality for as long as possible and dealing with it poorly when we can't deny it any longer. Responding to Nuland's observation, Barnes comments, "This is good news in one major sense—doctors are against death; less good in that they may unknowingly transfer their own fears on to their patients, over-insist on curability, and shun death as failure."

We have an idea about what is important to make death as good as it can be, given a process of dying that is sufficiently long (as is often the case for people with terminal cancers). The things that are important to the one doing the dying are surprisingly ordinary and easy to accomplish. Karen Steinhauser and colleagues questioned 1,500 people, including seriously ill patients, recently bereaved families, physicians, nurses, social workers, clergy members, and hospice volunteers. More than 70 percent considered the same ten things most important while dying. In rank order they were to 1) be kept clean, 2) name a decision maker, 3) have a nurse with whom one feels comfortable, 4) know what to expect about one's physical condition, 5) have someone who will listen, 6) maintain one's dignity, 7) trust one's physician, 8) have one's financial affairs in order, 9) be free of pain, and 10) maintain a sense of humor. Those seem like pretty minimal deathbed requests. The growing specialty of palliative care and the hospice movement are making strides toward granting those requests for people for whom the process of dying is long, helping to make for them a death as good as it can be.

But dying for many Americans does not happen in the peaceful and caring confines of a hospice or at home surrounded by loved ones. More than 20 percent of dying Americans spend their last days in an expensive, high-tech hospital intensive care unit. A report from the National Bureau of Economic Research estimates that the cost of the final year of life consumes a "substantial fraction of liquid wealth for decedents." In an episode of *60 Minutes* ("The Cost of Dying") in 2009, Ira Byock, a physician at New Hampshire's Dartmouth-Hitchcock Medical Center, told reporter Steve Kroft: "This is not the way most people would want to spend the last days of their life. And yet this has become almost the medical last rites for people as they die." He added that "denial of death at some point becomes a delusion, and we start acting in ways that make no sense whatsoever." Although most Americans say they want to die at home, 75 percent of us die in a hospital or nursing home.

Carleton Hensley may have been fortunate to spend his final days in a hospital before the advent of technologically sophisticated intensive care units. There were many unpleasant things about his dying, but he had the advantage of doing it while holding the hand of his devoted wife, their terminal intimacies unimpeded by a breathing tube and a ventilator. Everything that modern critical care medicine could have provided him might have forestalled the inevitable for a few days, even a week or two, but would not have altered the outcome.

Given that we are all destined to share the same eventual fate, one would think that we would deal with that inevitability with more grace. And if, as the time nears, we have our wits, we suspect that, absent social pressures to the contrary, we would eschew the technical heroics in favor of peace with ourselves and those we care about. But our medical system often fosters social pressures to the contrary. Physicians need to tell a dying person's loved ones, "We did all we could," probably more than loved ones need to hear it. Did all you could to what? Thwart the natural course of things? The medical profession's preoccupation with immortality, our capacity for denying the inevitability of the grim reaper's visitation, uses up a lot of resources, both monetary and emotional, that could be put to better use. The proliferation of drugs and devices that can postpone the inevitable for a bit often tempts us to avoid confronting our mortality until it is too late to deal with it constructively. I cannot confront my fate from the depths of a drug-induced coma while assaulted by machines that make me breathe when all the forces of my nature resist and drugs that flog my failing heart to exhaustion. Dying that way doesn't do much to comfort those from whom I am taking my final leave, either.

This is not to say that high-tech medicine doesn't have a place. Intensive care units and the sophisticated care delivered there save the lives of people who would otherwise die. That is even true for the elderly who have reversible disease. But it is neither the right nor in the best interest of everyone who is entering their terminal days to spend them in an ICU.

The Institute of Medicine defines a good death as "one that is free from avoidable death and suffering for patients, families and caregivers in general accordance with the patients' and families' wishes." That institution and several others, including the Robert Wood Johnson Foundation, have studied the topic, produced reports that document failures of the medical profession, and called for change in how we deal with death. But old habits die hard. We still have much to learn about our mortality and how to deal with it.

The Festa de Nossa Senhora da Boa Morte begins each year on the Friday closest to August 15 in the state of Bahia, Brazil, and lasts for three days. The festival is organized by the Irmande da Boa Morte (Sisterhood of the Good Death) and is a celebration of dance and prayer by descendants of African slaves in praise of their liberation. A procession of brilliantly clad Afro-Brazilian women wends through the narrow streets of Cachoeira along the Paraguacu River. They form a circle and dance the *samba-de-roda*. There is a cortege commemorating the death of Our Lady and a burial procession of Our Lady of the Good Death. There are food, music, and dancing for as long as the money holds out. This veneration of Our Lady of the Good Death was born from slavery, a way of defending individual value and honoring life. The sisterhood finds in a contemplation of the good death a celebration of a vibrant and joyful life. We can learn a lot from how others understand and deal with our shared mortality.

People have not always viewed the fact that we enter this life with an expiration date so negatively. More than two millennia ago, the Greek philosopher Epicurus argued that living well and dying well were essentially the same. Though he had other interesting ideas about living and dying well that have fueled controversy through the millennia, he at least was not haunted by a fear of dying. When his time came at the age of seventy-two, he wrote to Idomeneus, "I have written this letter to you on a happy day to me, which is also the last day of my life . . . the cheerfulness of my mind, which comes from the recollection of all my philosophical contemplation, counterbalances all these afflictions." Remembering a life that he perceived as well-lived brought him peace in dying.

Imminent death or the threat of it has a way of focusing one's attention. A potentially terminal experience (stroke, heart attack, a diagnosis of cancer) is a potent motivator for reviewing one's life and priorities. And priorities get rearranged. Such experiences are often life-changing. We start regretting all those hours we spent away from our families, the missed kids' ball games and dance recitals, time spent away from those we claim to value above all else while we were striving to make money, get promoted, be successful. Definitions of success change when it becomes impossible any longer to perpetuate the self-delusion of immortality (an adolescent delusion that we cling to until forced to give it up). We begin thinking about our legacy. What will we leave behind that has any value or durability? What is life about, anyway? Where did the time go? The brevity of the life experience impresses us when the dark at the end of the tunnel looms.

Life *is* brief. Hilda Echt lived more than a century, saw her kids finish careers and retire. But even at a hundred she wasn't ready to die. "I want to drop dead," she said, "but not yet!" She had done a lot, but there was more she wanted to do. She wanted more time. Any outside observer would describe her life as long, but a century didn't seem that long to her. No matter how long we live, life is brief. A hundred years? Some have speculated that a 120 might not be beyond possibility as we learn how to live healthier. Still a picosecond in historical time. In a sense longevity is an impossible illusion. We will never live all that long. Obsolescence is integral to our biology.

Sometimes life is very short. How people choose to deal with that brevity is interesting. Randolph Frederick "Randy" Pausch died of pancreatic cancer on July 25, 2008, at age forty-seven. When the diagnosis was made in August 2007, his doctors guessed he had three to six months of reasonable health left. How he spent those last months is a matter of extensive record in the popular press, on YouTube, and in numerous other places.

There was a lecture series at Carnegie Mellon, where Pausch was a professor, that asked noted academics to give a hypothetical "final talk." They were supposed to search themselves for what really mattered to them personally and try to present the results of their contemplation to an audience. Dr. Pausch took the podium before an audience of four hundred colleagues and students on September 18, 2007, a month or so after his diagnosis. After quieting a prolonged standing ovation from the audience he proceeded to deliver his lecture, "Really Achieving Your Childhood Dreams," punctuating a discourse on science education and his own life lessons with humor and an occasional set of push-ups. (Commenting on the recent change of the name of the lecture series from "Last Lecture" to "Journeys," he quipped, "I thought, damn, I finally nailed the venue and they renamed it.") A book based on his lecture became an immediate *New York Times* best seller. He spent his final months lobbying for causes he valued and doing some other things he had always wanted to do. Pausch inspired a lot of people to aim higher, to be better. It is quite likely that his legacy was magnified rather than diminished by the brevity of his life.

Why must we wait for a near fatal stroke, heart attack, or a fatal cancer to come to grips with the fact that we will die? How would we live if we experienced our mortality, realized how short the time is and how sure the final outcome, before being faced with an incapacitating illness? It seems likely that such a realization, internalized, would trigger some rearranging of priorities for most of us. And the reality of an inescapable end to what will be a too-brief life no matter when it ends could be liberating. "It's the soul afraid of dying who cannot learn to live," Bette Midler haunts with that line from *The Rose*. Perhaps the Angel of Death and the Angel of Mercy, like the "Colonel's Lady an' Judy O'Grady," in Kipling's poem, "are sisters under their skins!"

If we are to live as well as humanly possible, we are going to have to deal with this inevitability of death, as a personal experience, but also deal with our shared mortality as a social phenomenon. The surest prediction of Predictive Health is that every one of us will die. We don't need to sequence our genomes to be completely confident of that. We, that is those of us who have chosen to take on the responsibility of dealing with human health as a profession, are not doing very well in this area. Given any possible option, we avoid engaging the subject in any meaningful way. And we bear responsibility for disseminating that attitude to those we claim to serve. Death scares us nearly to death.

We must do better than that. If we choose to draw a battle line between the Grim Reaper's territory and that of human health care, we have engaged in a battle that we are destined to lose. If we can get over our fright at the prospect, understand that living and dying are not only part of the same continuum but, done well, are integral to each other, we will change how we approach our own mortality and that of those for whom we care. Although we won't abolish the specialty of critical care or the ICUs where that specialty is acted out, a lot of people who die there now will die a better death somewhere else.

Life is a fatal condition. Make the best of it.

Notes

Chapter 1: Ponce's Dream

5   **health care within a decade or so:** Lee Hood outlines his vision of personalized medicine for the next ten years, *Nature Biotechnology* 29 (2011): 191–193.

Chapter 3: Toward Exemplary Health

19   **poem are equally valid for present-day medicine:** Blind men and an elephant, *Wikipedia*, http://en.wikipedia.org/wiki/Blind_men_and _an_elephant; John Godfrey Saxe, The blind men and the elephant, http://constitution.org/col/blind_men.htm.

19   **"merely the absence of disease or infirmity":** Preamble to the Constitution of the World Health Organization as adopted by the International Health Conference, New York, June 1946, signed on July 22, 1946, by the representatives of sixty-one states and entered into force on April 7, 1948. Official Records of the WHPO, no. 2: 100.

19   **report ushered in the modern medical era:** Abraham Flexner, Medical education in the United States: A report to the Carnegie Foundation for the Advancement of Teaching, Bulletin no. 4 (1910); Flexner report, *Wikipedia*, http://en.wikipedia.org/wiki/Flexner _Report.

21   **"prate about the elephant not one of [us] has seen":** Saxe, The blind men and the elephant.

22   **of otherwise similar people without that stress:** A. Damjanovic, Y. Yang, R. Glaser, J. Kiecolt-Glaser, H. Nguyen, B. Laskowski, Y. Zou, D. Beversdorf, and N. Weng, Accelerated telomere erosion

is associated with declining immune function of caregivers of Alzheimer's disease patients, *Journal of Immunology* 179 (2007): 4249–4254.

22 **as treatment for cancer often became depressed:** A. Miller and C. Raison, Immune system contributions to the pathophysiology of depression, *FOCUS* 6 (2008): 36–45.

24 **"a state of *complete* physical, mental and social well-being":** Preamble to the Constitution of the World Health Organization.

24 **the other end by the opposite condition, *languishing*:** C. Keyes and K. Haidt, eds., *Flourishing: Positive psychology and the life well lived* (Washington, DC: American Psychological Association, 2003).

26 **comes from studies of men in Sweden:** L. Welin, K. Scardsudd, S. Ander-Peciva, G. Tibblin, B. Tibblin, and B. Larsson, Prospective study of social influences on mortality, *The Lancet*, April 20, 1985.

Chapter 4: Health in the Age of the Omics

29 *of God* **and** *The Language of Life*: Francis Collins, *The language of life: DNA and the revolution in personalized medicine* (New York: HarperCollins, 2010).

30 **was much lower, more like twenty thousand:** Human genome project, http://www.ornl.gov/sci/techresources/Human_Genome/home.shtml.

31 **assembled in twenty thousand different sequences:** Human genome project.

31 **the language of life are astoundingly simple:** Human genome project.

31 **"most, if not all, human diseases":** Declan Butler, Science after the sequence, *Nature* 465 (2010): 1000–1001.

33 **"medicine has not been well quantified":** W. G. Feero, A. E. Guttmacher, and F. S. Collins, Genomic medicine: An updated primer, *New England Journal of Medicine* 362 (2010): 2001–2011.

33 **"Genomics is a way to do science not medicine":** Nicholas Wade, A decade later, genetic map yields few new cures, *New York Times*, June 12, 2010.

33 **these genetic copies make up the transcriptome:** Feero, Guttmacher, and Collins, Genomic medicine.

35   that carry out the vital life processes: G. Marko-Varga and E.
     Fehniger, Proteomics and disease—the challenges for technology
     and discovery, *Journal of Proteome Research* 3 (2004): 167–178.

35   well before it happens: Metabolomics: Signs of a long life, *The
     Economist*, June 20, 2008.

36   an individual's unique metabolic profile: Metabolomics.

Chapter 5: Taming the Wild Genome

41   orchestration of a sizable fraction of the genome: KAP Biology De-
     partment, Kenyon College, Chapter 11: Development: Differentia-
     tion and determination, http://biology.Kenyon.edu/courses/biol114
     /Chapter_11.htm.

42   "are not subject to 21 U.S.C. 343(r)(6)": Vasilios H. Frankos, PhD,
     Director, Division of Dietary Supplement Programs, FDA, to
     Dennis Jones, PhD, Somalabs, Inc., http://www.regulations.gov
     /#!documentDetail;D=FDA-1997-S-0006-1032.

42   "prevent, mitigate or cure chronic disease": J. Kaput and R. L. Ro-
     driguez, Nutritional genomics: The next frontier in the postge-
     nomic era, *Physiological Genomics* 16 (2004): 166–177.

43   anything else in their diet: S. H. Zeisel, Is there a new component
     of the Mediterranean diet that reduces inflammation? *American
     Journal of Clinical Nutrition* 87 (2008): 277–278.

44   Michael Pollan's "eat less, mostly plants": Michael Pollan, *The om-
     nivore's dilemma: A natural history of four meals* (New York: Penguin
     Press, 2006).

44   relevant to systemic health: F. W. Booth, M. V. Chakavarthy, and
     E. E. Spangerburg, Exercise and gene expression: Physiological reg-
     ulation of the human genome through physical activity, *Journal of
     Physiology* 543 (2002): 399–411; F. W. Booth and P. D. Neufer,
     Exercise controls gene expression, *American Scientist* 93 (2005):
     28–35.

45   stereotype is not a biological phenomenon: C. W. Cotman and
     N. C. Berchtold, Exercise: A behavioral intervention to enhance brain
     health and plasticity, *Trends in Neuroscience* 25 (2002): 295–301.

45   cell-to-cell communication: T. Hayashi, O. Urayama, K. Kawai,
     K. Hayashi, S. Iwanaga, M. Ohta, T. Saito, and K. Murakami,

Laughter regulates gene expression in patients with type 2 diabetes, *Psychotherapy and Psychosomatics* 75 (2006): 106.

45 **underexpressed ones suggested decreased resistance to infection:** Randall Parker, Lonely people have different gene expression patterns, *FuturePundit: Brain Emotions Archives*, September 12, 2007, http://www.futurepundit.com/archives/cat_brain_emotions.html.

46 **Only 3 percent of mammalian species are monogamous:** Sylvia Wrobel, Coupling: Monogamy—vole style, *Emory Health* 3 (Spring 2010): 3–6.

47 **very different and in opposite directions:** S. Sajikumar, S. Navakkode, V. Korz, and J. Frey, Cognitive and emotional information processing: Protein synthesis and gene expression, *Journal of Physiology* 584, no. 2 (2007): 389–400.

47 **398 residents of various regions of Flanders:** D. M. van Leeuwen, R. W. H. Gottschalk, G. Schoeters, N. A. van Larebeke, V. Nelen, W. F. Baeyens, J. C. S. Kleinjans, and J. H. M. van Delft, Transcriptome analysis in peripheral blood of humans exposed to environmental carcinogens: A promising new biomarker in environmental health studies, *Environmental Health Perspectives* 116 (2008): 1519–1525.

Chapter 6: The Epigenome

50 **major effects on how it functions:** Epigenetics, *Wikipedia,* http://enwikipedia.org/wiki/Epigenetics.

50 **meaning above or in addition to genetics:** Epigenetics.

51 **each successive generation of a specific organ's cells:** Epigenetics; In their nurture, *Nature* 467, no. 9 (2010): 146–148.

51 **(e.g., their fingerprints are slightly different):** Do identical twins have the same fingerprints? *Health,* September 30, 2009, http://earthsky.org/health/identical-twins-fingerprint.

51 **identical twins may have very different personalities:** Nicholas Wade, Explaining differences in twins, *New York Times,* July 5, 2005; Chris Mooney, Of twins and centenarians, *Sage Crossroads,* June 30, 2003, http://www.sagecrossroads.net/node/331; Do identical twins have the same fingerprints?; Sarah Pierce, Why do iden-

tical twins have physical differences if they have the same DNA? *Understanding Genetics*, September 16, 2005, http://www.thetech .org/genetics/ask.php?id=142.

52 **different health and medical histories:** Wade, Explaining differences in twins.

53 **from some cancers to obesity to diabetes:** Pete Myers, Good genes gone bad, *The American Prospect*, March 19, 2006; Bette Hileman, Chemicals can turn genes on and off; new tests needed, scientists say, *Environmental Health News*, August 3, 2009.

54 **deal with our planet and its component parts:** Myers, Good genes gone bad; Hileman, Chemicals can turn genes on and off.

54 **affected by what a pregnant mother eats:** D. C. Dolinoy, J. R. Weidman, and R. L. Jirtle, Epigenetic gene regulation: Linking early developmental environment to adult disease, *Reproductive Toxicology* 23 (2007): 297–307; Kate Travis, Eat your way to a better DNA, *The Scientist* 20 (2006): 50.

55 **just like the rats from the better homes:** Hileman, Chemicals can turn genes on and off.

55 **so that they no longer act like cancer:** Hileman, Chemicals can turn genes on and off.

Chapter 7: Biomarkers and Biobanks

57 **cheek lining should be enough to find them:** Wellcome Trust, Briefing: From biobanks to biomarkers, www.wellcome.ac.uk /publications.

58 **enough sensitivity to predict impending dysfunctions:** Lee Hood outlines his vision of personalized medicine for the next 10 years, *Nature Biotechnology* 29 (2011): 191–193.

60 **most of the common human diseases:** Gary Stix, Is chronic inflammation the key to unlocking the mysteries of cancer? *Scientific American* (July 2007); Autoimmunity, *Wikipedia*, http://en.wikipedia .org/wiki/Autoimmunity; R. Wayne Alexander, Hypertension and the pathogenesis of atherosclerosis: Oxidative stress and the mediation of arterial inflammatory response: A new perspective, *Hypertension* 25 (1995): 155–161.

60   invasion by the real-world culprit: Autoimmunity.

61   the victim's most vulnerable organ(s): Stix, Is chronic inflamma-
       tion the key; Autoimmunity; Alexander, Hypertension and the
       pathogenesis of atherosclerosis.

62   the healthier we are: V. Schachinger and A. M. Zeiher, Stem cells and
       cardiovascular and renal disease: Today and tomorrow, *Journal of
       the American Society of Nephrology* 16 (2005): S2–S6; A. Atala, R.
       Lanza, J. Thomson, and R. Nerem, *Principles of regenerative medicine*
       (Burlington, MA: Academic Press, 2008); J. M. Hill, G. Zalos, J. P.
       J. Halcox, W. H. Schenke, M. A. Waclawiw, A. A. Quyyumi, and T.
       Finkel, Circulating endothelial progenitor cells, vascular function, and
       cardiovascular risk, *New England Journal of Medicine* 348 (2003): 7.

62   it as FACS for obvious reasons: Hill et al., Circulating endothelial
       progenitor cells.

62   in addition to the heart and blood vessels: Schachinger and Zeiher,
       Stem cells and cardiovascular and renal disease; Atala et al., *Princi-
       ples of regenerative medicine.*

63   similar dysfunctions of fundamental processes: F. Sofi, R. Abbate,
       G. F. Gensini, and A. Casini, Accruing evidence on benefits of ad-
       herence to the Mediterranean diet on health: An updated system-
       atic review and meta-analysis, *American Journal of Clinical Nutrition*
       92 (2010): 1189–1196.

63   but doesn't know which half: N. B. Giuse, Riding the waves of
       change together: Are we all paying attention? *Journal of the Medical
       Library Association* 96 (2008): 85–87.

63   the times and locations of their visits: Wellcome Trust, Briefing.

64   the overall bill may approach £10 billion: UK scientist blasts
       biobank project, *BioNews* 274, http://www.bionews.org.uk/page
       _12097.asp.

64   that country's national health system: Gisli Palsson, The rise and
       fall of a biobank: The case of Iceland, *Biobanks* 17 (2008): 41.

65   grant from the National Institutes of Health: D. M. Roden, J. M.
       Pulley, M. A. Basford, G. R. Bernard, E. W. Clayton, J. R. Balser,
       and D. R. Masys, Development of a large-scale de-identified DNA
       biobank to enable personalized medicine, *Clinical Pharmacology &
       Therapeutics* 84 (2008): 362–369.

67   Like Thomas Friedman's world: T. L. Friedman, *The world is flat* (New York: Farrar, Straus & Giroux, 2005).

Chapter 8: Zip Codes and Genetic Codes

69   than if you live in southern California: R. J. Eisen, R. S. Lane, C. I. Fritz, and L. Eisen, Spatial patterns of Lyme disease risk in California based on disease incidence data and modeling of vector-tick exposure, *American Journal of Tropical Medicine & Hygiene* 75 (2006): 669–676.

70   South Dakota town with a high mix use index: J. S. Marks, Why your zip code may be more important to your health than your genetic code, *Huffington Post*, April 23, 2009, http://www.huffington post.com/james-marks/why-your-zip-code-may-be_b_190650 .html; L. R. Mobley, E. D. Root, E. A. Finkelstein, O. Khavjou, R. P. Farris, and J. C. Will, Environment, obesity, and cardiovascular disease risk in low-income women, *American Journal of Preventive Medicine* 30 (2006): 327–332.

71   not attributes of specific people: D. A. Henderson and F. D. Scutchfield, Point-counterpoint: The public health versus medical model of prevention, *American Journal of Preventive Medicine* 5 (1989): 113–119.

72   all the doctors in the city: John Snow (Physician), *Wikipedia*, http://en.wikipedia.org/wiki/John_Snow_(physician).

73   *"the probability of a single event is a meaningless concept"*: Steven Pinker, My genome, my self, *New York Times Magazine*, January 7, 2009.

74   actually lived a very long time: Stephen Jay Gould, The median isn't the message, http://www.cancerguide.org/median_not_msg.html.

74   "actual world of variations, shadings and continua": Gould, The median isn't the message.

Chapter 9: Cyberhealth/Technohealth

77   handle about seven things at a time: The Blue Ridge Academic Health Group, Advancing value in health care: The emerging transformational role of informatics, Report 12, October 2008,

http://whsc.emory.edu/blueridge/_pdf/blue_ridge_report>12
>2008.pdf.

77 **"systems, understanding and technology":** Blue Ridge Academic
Health Group, Advancing value in health care.

77 **doubles roughly every two years:** Moore's Law, *Wikipedia*,
http://en.wikipedia.org/wiki/Moore's_law.

79 **number is undoubtedly much larger now:** James G. Anderson and
Kenneth Goodman, *Ethics and information technology* (New York:
Springer Verlag, 2002).

81 **Does that make any difference?:** A. K. Jha, J. B. Perlin, K. W.
Kizer, and R. A. Dudley, Effect of the transformation of the Veterans Affairs Health Care System on the quality of care, *New England Journal of Medicine* 348, no. 22 (2003): 2218–2227.

81 **organization in the country that would like to use it:** VistA,
Wikipedia, http://en.wikipedia.org/wiki/VistA.

82 **to remedy that with a new, compatible system:** Department of Defense and Department of Veterans Affairs, *Good News* 3, no. 1,
http://www.tricare.mil/DVPCO/downloads/DoD%20and%20VA
%20Good%20News%20Volume%203%20Issue%201.pdf.

82 **in all of history up to 2003:** E. Schmidt, Every 2 days we create as
much information as we did up to 2003, TechCrunch, August 4,
2010, http://techcrunch.com/2010/08/04/schmidt-data/.

83 **puts the problem this way:** E. O. Voit and K. L. Brigham, The role
of systems biology in predictive health and personalized medicine,
The Open Pathology Journal 2 (2008): 68–70.

84 **personalized, preemptive, and participatory:** L. Hood, A vision for
personalized medicine, *Technology Review*, March 9, 2010, http://
www.technologyreview.com/biomedicine/24703/.

85 **local pharmacy, and a computer:** SoloHealth, http://solohealth.com/.

Chapter 10: Truth and Consequences

89 **"You can see a lot just by looking":** Y. Berra, http://www.quote
world.org/quotes/12139.

90 **"but in having new eyes":** M. Proust, http://thinkexist.com/quotes
/marcel_proust/.

90 *Novum Organum,* **published in 1620:** M. Heese, Francis Bacon's philosophy of science, in *Essential articles for the study of Francis Bacon,* ed. Brian Vickers (Hamden, CT: Archon Books, 1968), 114–139.

90 **followed by experiment:** A. Carpi, The scientific method, http://web.jjay.cuny.edu/~acarpi/NSC/1-scimethod.htm.

90 **which regulates blood sugar:** Nobelprize.org, Diabetes and insulin: The discovery of insulin, http://www.nobelprize.org/educational/medicine/insulin/discovery-insulin.html.

92 **details of the family histories:** J. H. Newman, L. Wheeler, K. B. Lane, E. Loyd, R. Gaddapati, J. A. Phillips, and J. E. Loyd, Mutation in the gene for bone morphogenetic protein receptor II as a cause of primary pulmonary hypertension in a large kindred, *New England Journal of Medicine* 345 (2001): 319–324.

93 **"the point is to discover them":** Galileo Galilei, *Wikiquotes,* http://en.wikiquote.org/wiki/Galileo_Galilei.

93 **Comroe called his research on research:** Julius H. Comroe, *Exploring the heart: Discoveries in heart disease and high blood pressure* (New York: W.W. Norton, Co., 1984).

94 **thought of making such machines:** Comroe, *Exploring the heart.*

95 **expanded upon in a book by that title:** Donald Stokes, *Pasteur's quadrant: Basic science and technological innovation* (Washington, DC: The Brookings Institution, 1997).

98 **public sphere and the world of commerce:** J. A. Henderson and J. J. Smith, Academia, industry, and the Bayh-Dole Act: An implied duty to commercialize (October 2002): 1–9, http://www.cimit.org/news/regulatory/coi_part3.pdf.

Chapter 11: Resonance

99 **"in practice they are not":** A. Einstein, http://www.goodreads.com/quotes/show/66864; Diplomacy, *Wikipedia,* http://en.wikipedia.org/wiki/Diplomacy.

100 **"in me more than most other men":** Antony van Leeuwenhoek (1632–1723), http://www.ucmp.berkeley.edu/history/leeuwenhoek.html.

101 **"so miserable that life seemed worthless"/he set about to understand and change it:** O. Hanninen, M. Farago, and E. Monnos,

Ignatz Philipp Semmelweis, the prophet of bacteriology, *Infection Control* 4 (1983): 367–370; S. B. Nuland, *The doctors' plague: Germs, childbed fever and the strange story of Ignac Semmelweis* (New York: W.W. Norton, 2003); Ignaz Semmelweis, *Etiology, concept and prophylaxis of childbed fever* (Madison: University of Wisconsin Press, 1983).

102 **Mason Academy of Medicine in Middleport, Ohio:** George Huntington, *Wikipedia*, http://en.wikipedia.org/wiki/George_Huntington.

103 **only two scientific publications during his career:** G. Huntington, On chorea, *Medical and Surgical Reporter of Philadelphia* 26 (1872): 317–321.

103 **"more graphically or more briefly described":** Huntington's disease, *Wikipedia*, http://en.wikipedia.org/wiki/Huntington's_disease.

103 **at Royal Perth Hospital in 1979:** Barry Marshall, *Wikipedia*, http://en.wikipedia.org/wiki/Barry_Marshall.

104 **but an obsession nonetheless:** B. Marshall, Helicobacter connections, Nobel lecture, December 8, 2005, http://nobelprize.org/nobel_prizes/medicine/laureates/2005/marshall-lecture.html.

104 **Robert Koch and Friedrich Loeffler in the late nineteenth century:** J. Grimes, Koch's postulates: Then and now, *Microbe* (May 2006), http://forms.asm.org/microbe/index.asp?bid=42390.

Chapter 12: The Devils We Know

110 **obesity and its associated ills:** Ken Thorpe, C. Florence, D. Howard, and P. Joski, Trends: The impact of obesity on rising medical spending, *Health Affairs* (2004). doi: 10.1377/hlthaff.w4.480.

111 **a species that can eat anything:** Michael Pollan, *The omnivore's dilemma: A natural history of four meals* (New York: Penguin Press, 2006).

111 **the genesis of the epidemic:** George J. Armelagos, The omnivore's dilemma: The evolution of the brain and the determinants of food choice, *Journal of Anthropological Research* 66 (2010): 161–186.

112 **we have simply outpaced our genes:** Greg Gibson, *It takes a genome: How a clash between our genes and modern life is making us*

sick (Upper Saddle River, NJ: Pearson Education Inc., FT Press Science, 2009).

113 **a major explanation for the problem:** Gina Kolata, *Rethinking thin: The new science of weight loss—and the myths and realities of dieting* (New York: Farrar, Straus & Giroux, 2007).

114 **much as they would do in the wild:** Yerkes National Primate Research Center, http://www.yerkes.emory.edu/.

115 **not body weight or BMI, is the culprit:** The scales can lie: Hidden fat, *The Wall Street Journal*, January 26, 2010.

116 **mentally, socially, physically, and spiritually:** K. L. Brigham, Predictive health: The coming revolution in health care, *Journal of the American Geriatric Society* 58, supp. 2 (2010): S298–S302.

117 **fat metabolism was immediately increased:** Gretchen Reynolds, A workout for your bloodstream, *New York Times Magazine,* June 20, 2010.

Chapter 13: Evidence-Based Health

120 **a relatively recent concept:** A. L. Cochrane, *Effectiveness and efficiency: Random reflections on health services* (London: Nuffield Provincial Hospitals Trust, 1972; reprinted in 1989 in association with the *BMJ*; reprinted in 1999 for Nuffield Trust by the Royal Society of Medicine Press, London); Evidence-Based Medicine Working Group, Evidence-based medicine: A new approach to teaching the practice of medicine, *JAMA* 268 (1992): 2420–2425.

121 **more research on the reviewed topic:** D. M. El Dib, A. N. Atallah, and R. B. Andriolo, Mapping the Cochrane evidence for decision making in health care, *Journal of Evaluation in Clinical Practice* 13 (2007): 689–692; The Cochrane Collaboration, http://www .cochrane.org/about-us/evidence-based-health-care.

122 **"descriptive studies, or reports of committees":** Evidence-based medicine, *Wikipedia*, http://en.wikipedia.org/wiki/Evidence-based _medicine.

122 **"experience and the best external evidence":** D. L. Sackett, W. M. Rosenberg, J. A. Gray, R. B. Haynes, and W. S. Richardson,

Evidence based medicine: What is it is and what it isn't, *British Medical Journal* 312 (1996): 71–72.

123 **taken as a supplement to them:** S. L. DeFelice, FIM rationale and proposed guidelines for the Nutraceutical Research & Education Act-NREA, November 10, 2002, Foundation for Innovation in Medicine, http://www.fimdefelice.org/archives/arc.researchact.html.

125 **could not possibly have contained any antibodies:** E. Dayenas, F. Beauvais, J. Amara, M. Oberbaum, B. Robinzon, A. Miadonna, A. Tedeschit, B. Pomeranz, P. Fortner, P. Belon, J. Sainte-Laudy, B. Poitevin, and J. Benveniste, Human basophil degranulation triggered by very dilute antiserum against IgE, *Nature* 333 (1988): 816–818.

125 **replicated in the tube with only water:** A. Coghlan, Scorn over claim of teleported DNA, *New Scientist,* January 12, 2011, 1–4.

125 **patients in intensive care units:** M. Frass, C. Dielacher, M. Linkesch, C. Endler, I. Muchitsch, E. Schuster, and A. Kaye, Influence of potassium dichromate on tracheal secretions in critically ill patients, *Chest* 127 (2005): 936–941.

126 **may even have clinically important effects:** H. K. Beecher, The powerful placebo, *JAMA* 159 (1955): 1602–1606.

126 **Hawthorne effect as the explanation:** A. Hrobjartsson and P. C. Gotzche. Placebo interventions for all clinical conditions, *Cochrane Database System Review* 106, no. 1: CD003974, http://www.ncbi .nlm.nih.gov/pubmed/20091554.

127 **the body's response to psychosocial stress:** T. W. W. Pace, L. T. Negi, D. D. Adame, S. P. Cole, T. I. Sivilli, T. D. Brown, M. J. Issa, and C. L. Raison, Effect of compassion meditation on neuroendocrine, innate immune and behavioral responses to psychosocial stress, *Psychoneuroendocrinology* 34 (2009): 87–98.

Chapter 14: Good Drugs

129 **a conversation about Predictive Health:** M. Terrezas, Future holds a lot for forum panelists, *Emory Report* 58, no. 27 (April 18, 2005).

130 **the Life Extension Buyers Club:** Life Extension Foundation, Top ten life extension drugs, http://www.esculape.com/bricabrac/topten lifeextensiondrugs.html.

130   **list of so-called immune-enhancing pills:** Doc's Pharmacy, Vitamin and herbal supplements from Doc's, http://www.docsdrugs.com/vitamins.asp; StemEnhance™ adult stem cell enhancement, http://www.astrologyzine.com/stemtech-stemenhance-stem-cell-enhancer-shtml; ActivaMune immune support formula, http://www.activamune.com/?gclid=CIu-kJyf7KYCFYXD7QodsVWdGQ.

133   **drugs to affect stem cells:** A stem-cell-boosting drug goes to clinical trial, Children's Hospital Boston, http://stemcell.childrenshospital.org/treating-patients/a-stem-cell-boosting-drug-goes-from-fishtank-to-bedside-2/.

133   **just like exercise:** E. Singer, New drugs mimic exercise, *Technology Review: Biomedicine* (July 31, 2008), http://www.technologyreview.com/biomedicine/21154/?a=f; J. Keeley, Researchers identify drugs that enhance exercise endurance, July 28, 2008, http://www.eurekalert.org/pub_releases/2008-07/hhmi-rid072808.php.

134   **exercise without the work:** E. Singer, New drugs mimic exercise.

Chapter 15: Disrupting Medical Care

138   **disruptive innovations in health care in books and journal articles:** C. M. Christensen, R. Bohmer, and J. Kenagy, Will disruptive innovations cure health care? *Harvard Business Review* (September–October 2000): 1–10.

139   **"sophisticated things in less expensive settings":** C. M. Christensen, J. H. Grossman, and J. Hwang, *The innovator's prescription: A disruptive solution for health care* (New York: McGraw Hill, 2009).

141   **"how people evaluate their lives":** E. Diener, S. Oishi, and R. E. Lucas, Personality, culture and subjective well-being: emotional and cognitive evaluations of life, *Annual Review of Psychology* 54 (2003): 403–425.

141   **determined to spread the word:** Penny George Institute for Health and Healing, http://www.bravewell.org/patient_empowerment/bravewell_clinical_network/institute_health_healing/.

142   **from many parts of the facility:** Duke Integrative Medicine, http://www.dukeintegrativemedicine.org/; Scripps Center for

Integrative Medicine, http://www.scripps.org/services/integrative
-medicine.

146   **means for combining social media and health care:** Centers for
Disease Control and Prevention, CDC GIS Web applications,
http://www.cdc.gov/gis/applications.htm; Mayo Clinic Social Media
Health Network, http://socialmedia.mayoclinic.org/network/.

147   **"in ways that lead to better health":** Go viral to improve health,
IOM-NAE Health Data Collegiate Challenge, http://iom.edu
/Activities/PublicHealth/GoViral.aspx.

147   **individual's risk for obesity than genetics:** N. A. Christakis and J. H.
Fowler, The spread of obesity in a large social network over 32
years, *New England Journal of Medicine* 357 (2007): 370–379.

149   **thinks he or she told them to do:** J. J. Vlasnik, S. L. Aliotta, and
B. DeLor, Medication adherence: Factors influencing compliance
with prescribed medication plans, *Case Manager* 16 (2005): 47–51;
R. A. Elliott and J. L. Marriott, Standardized assessment of patients'
capacity to manage medications: A systematic review of published
instruments, *BMC Geriatrics* 9 (2009): 27; R. M. Parker, D. W.
Baker, M. V. Williams, and J. R. Nurss, The test of functional health
literacy in adults: A new instrument for measuring patients' literacy
skills, *Journal of General Internal Medicine* 10 (1995): 537–541.

150   **interviews with patients exploring that chasm:** Parker et al., The
test of functional health literacy in adults.

151   **head in a different direction:** J. Schoemaker, Life changing experiences, May 20, 2009, http://www.shoemoney.com/2009/05/20
/life-changing-experiences/; S. Goldberg, What does it take for
events to change our behavior? Insights from the Chilean mine rescue, September 11th, and the global economic downturn, *Life as a
Human,* November 14, 2010, http://lifeasahuman.com/2010/current
-affairs/social-issues/what-does-it-take-for-events-to-change-our
-behavior-insights-from-the-chilean-mine-rescue-sept-11th-and
-the-global-economic-downturn/.

151   **A stroke can be a life-changing event:** W. Hayes, Former Miss Ari-
zona tells about life-changing impact of strokes, *Thetowntalk.com,*
February 26, 2011, http://www.thetowntalk.com/article/20110226
/NEWS01/102260326.

152 **Those programs appear to work:** Melko, C. N., P. E. Terry, K. Camp, M. Xi, and M. L. Healey. Diabetes health coaching improves medication adherence: A pilot study. *American Journal of Lifestyle Medicine* 4 (2011): 187–194.

154 **less expensive than the system we have now:** Christensen et al., *The innovator's prescription.*

155 **putting numbers to these benefits:** HSI: An Emory Georgia Tech initiative, http://www.hsi.gatech.edu/people/profile.php?entry=231.

Chapter 16: The Tyranny of Paradigm

159 **"Like clouds they shape themselves and go":** The Literature Network, Alfred, Lord Tennyson, In memoriam A.H.H., http://www.online-literature.com/donne/718/.

159 **"And you are the one who'll decide where to go":** Dr. Seuss, *Oh the places you'll go* (New York: Random House, 1990).

160 **paradigms of the sort that Thomas Kuhn discussed:** T. S. Kuhn, *The structure of scientific revolutions*, 3rd ed. (Chicago and London: University of Chicago Press, 1996).

162 **an advisory committee on the subject, which he chaired:** J. T. White, Luther Leonidas Terry, in *The national cyclopedia of American biography*, Vol. M. (New York: James T. White & Company, 1978); Luther Terry (1911–1985), *Encyclopedia of Alabama*, http://www.encyclopediaofalabama.org/face/Article.jsp?id=h-1241; Luther Leonidas Terry, *Wikipedia*, http://en.wikipedia.org/wiki/Luther_Terry.

162 **Its impact, though not immediate, was profound:** *Smoking and health: Report of the Advisory Committee to the Surgeon General of the United States* (Washington, DC: U.S. Department of Health, Education and Welfare, Public Health Service, 1964).

162 **half as many Americans smoked in 2010 as did in 1964:** *Trends in current cigarette smoking among high school students and adults, United States, 1965–2010*, http://www.cdc.gov/tobacco/data_statistics/tables/trends/cig_smoking/index.htm.

163 **didn't understand the debate in December 2009:** Reynolds Staff, Pew study: Health-care reform coverage focused on politics, not

system, June 21, 2010, http://businessjournalism.org/2010/06/21/pew-study-health-care-reform-coverage-focused-on-politics-not-system.

164   **new approaches to customer service:** B. Menninger, Reinventing health care delivery: Innovation and improvement behind the scenes, *California Health Foundation Issue Brief* (September 2009): 1–14; Kaiser Permanente, Thrive, http://thrivewithkp.org.

164   **"than wait until the system collapses":** Reinventing health care delivery: Innovation and improvement behind the scenes, *California HealthCare Foundation Issue Brief* (September 2009): 1–13, http://www.chcf.org/~/media/MEDIA%20LIBRARY%20Files/PDF/I/PDF%20InnovationCenters.pdf.

164   **negative disease prevention approach:** Kaiser Permanente, Thrive.

164   **reviews some of those experiences:** L. L. Berry, A. M. Mirabito, and W. B. Baun, What's the hard return on employee wellness programs? *Harvard Business Review* (December 2010): 104–112.

165   **produced even more dramatic results:** Berry et al., What's the hard return on employee wellness programs?

165   **saving $1.5 million in paid sick leave:** Berry et al., What's the hard return on employee wellness programs?

167   **two different kinds of medical practice:** Flexner report, *Wikipedia,* http://en.wikipedia.org/wiki/Flexner_Report.

167   **document that changed the paradigm:** A. Flexner, *Medical education in the United States and Canada: A report to the Carnegie Foundation for the Advancement of Teaching,* Bulletin no. 4 (New York: The Carnegie Foundation for the Advancement of Teaching, 1910).

168   **"and well being and improve care":** Institute of Health and Biomedical Innovation, Queensland University of Technology, https://www.ihbi.qut.edu.au/.

169   **approaches to innovation in health care:** Center for Research on Health Care, University of Pittsburgh, http://www.crhc.pitt.edu/about.html.

169   **those centers are required to be interdisciplinary:** Clinical and Translational Science Awards, National Center for Research Resources, National Institutes of Health, http://www.ncrr.nih.gov/clinical_research_resources/clinical_and_translational_science_awards/.

170 **educational experiences for doctors in training:** H. K. Rabinowitz, D. Babbott, S. Bastacky, J. M. Pascoe, K. K. Patel, K. L. Pye, J. Rodak Jr., K. J. Veit, and D. L. Wood, Innovative approaches to educating medical students for practice in a changing health care environment: The National UME-21 Project, *Academic Medicine* 76 (2001): 587–597.

171 **bridge laboratory and population sciences:** Institutional Program Unifying Laboratory and Population Based Sciences, Burroughs Wellcome Fund, http://www.bwfund.org/pages/159/Institutional -Program-Unifying-Population-and-Laboratory-Based-Sciences/.

Chapter 17: Healthy People—Healthy Planet

175 **And the benefits were good:** D. Rudacille, *Roots of steel: Boom and bust in an American mill town* (New York: Pantheon Books, 2010); T. Bishop, The legacy of Sparrows Point: Steel mill, company town, center of community life, *Baltimore Sun,* August 5, 2007.

175 **"depends on his not understanding":** Upton Sinclair, *Wikiquote,* http://en.wikiquote.org/wiki/Upton_Sinclair.

176 **except for the events of October 27–31, 1948:** B. Roueche, The fog, *The New Yorker,* September 30, 1950; B. Roueche, *Eleven blue men* (New York: Little Brown, 1953).

176 **probably had its roots in Donora:** Donora, Pennsylvania, *Wikipedia,* http://en.wikipedia.org/wiki/Donora_Pennsylvania; Donora smog, *Wikipedia,* http://en.wikipedia.org/wiki/1948_Donora _smog; S. D. Hamill, Unveiling a museum, a Pennsylvania town remembers the smog that killed 20, *New York Times,* November 1, 2008.

177 **sickened thousands more:** J. J. Stegeman and A. R. Solow, A look back at the London Smog of 1952 and the half century since: A half century later: Recollections of the London Fog, *Environmental Health Perspectives* 110 (December 2002): a734–a735; The London Smog disaster of 1952: Days of toxic darkness, http://www .portfolio.mvm.ed.ac.uk/studentwebs/session4/27/greatsmog52.htm; R. Baldwin, The great London smog of 1952, *The Economist* 16 (August 20, 2008): 31.

177 which underlie most chronic illnesses: J. C. Chen and J. Schwartz, Metabolic syndrome and inflammatory responses to long-term particulate air pollutants, *Environmental Health Perspectives* 116 (2008): 612–617.

179 "each of us can make a difference": A. Gore, *An inconvenient truth: The planetary emergency of global warming and what we can do about it* (Emmaus, PA: Rodale Press, 2006).

180 "We think green means green": Quoted in Gore, *An inconvenient truth.*

180 "communion with the rest of creation": T. Roszak, *The voice of the earth: An exploration of ecopsychology* (Grand Rapids, MI: Phanes Press, 2002).

181 "intervention for populations": C. Maller, M. Townsend, A. Pryor, P. Brown, and L. St Leger, Healthy nature healthy people: "Contact with nature" as an upstream health promotion intervention for populations, *Health Promotion International* 21 (2005): 45–54.

181 "more than three of five deaths in Oregon": Healthy places, healthy people: A framework for Oregon, Health Promotion and Chronic Disease Prevention Program, Oregon Department of Human Services, Public Health Division, www.healthoregon.org/hpcdp.

Chapter 18: Toward a Square Wave Life

185 down to 70 or 80 in another decade: J. Flower, The future of healthcare, *Encyclopedia of the future* (New York: Macmillan and Co., 1996), http://www.well.com/~bbear/healthcare_future.html.

Epilogue

190 "'Because the universe is happening to you'": J. Barnes, *Nothing to be frightened of* (New York: Alfred A. Knopf, 2008).

190 denial, anger, bargaining, and depression: E. Kübler-Ross, *On death and dying* (New York: Routledge, 2008).

190 "personal anxieties about dying": Barnes, *Nothing to be frightened of.*

190 "and shun death as failure": Barnes, *Nothing to be frightened of.*

191   **maintain a sense of humor:** K. E. Steinhauser, E. C. Clipp, M. Mc-Neilly, et al., In search of a good death: Observations of patients, families and providers, *Annals of Internal Medicine* 132 (2000): 825–832.

191   **"substantial fraction of liquid wealth for decedents":** S. Marshall, K. M. McGarry, and J. S. Skinner, The risk of out-of-pocket health care expenditure at the end of life, National Bureau of Economic Research, Working paper no. 16170, July 2010, http://www.nber.org/papers/w16170.

191   **"that make no sense whatsoever":** The cost of dying: Patients' last two months of life cost Medicare $50 billion last year: Is there a better way? *60 Minutes,* CBS, November 19, 2009, http://www.cbsnews.com/stories/2009/11/19/60minutes/main5711689.shtml.

193   **"patients' and families' wishes":** D. H. Gustafson, A good death, *Journal of Medical Internet Research* 9 (2007): e6, http://www.jmir.org/2007/1/e6/.

193   **celebration of a vibrant and joyful life:** Sisterhood of the Good Death, *Feste Irmandade da Boa Morte,* http://salvadorbahiaguide.com/sisterhoodofthegooddeath.html.

194   **"counterbalances all these afflictions":** Epicurus letter to Idomeneus, www.epicurus.net.

195   **three to six months of reasonable health left:** Randy Pausch, *Wikipedia,* http://en.wikipedia.org/wiki/Randy_Pausch.

195   **immediate *New York Times* best seller:** R. Pausch, *The last lecture* (New York: Hyperion, 2008).

196   **"sisters under their skins!":** Rudyard Kipling, The ladies, http://www.everypoet.com/archive/poetry/Rudyard_Kipling/kipling_the_ladies.htm.

Additional Reading

Adams, S. Millions taking statin drugs "needlessly". *Cleaves Newswire*, January 26, 2011. http://cleaves.zapto.org/news/story-2296.html.

Adherence to long-term therapies: Evidence for action. Geneva: World Health Organization, 2003. http://www.who.int/chp/knowledge/publications /adherence_full_report.pdf.

American Cancer Society. Cancer information on the Internet. http://www .cancer.org/Cancer/CancerBasics/cancer-information-on-the-internet.

Ashish, K. J., C. M. DesRoches, E. G. Campbell, K. Donelan, S. R. Rao, T. G. Ferris, A. Shields, S. Rosenbaum, and D. Blumenthal. Use of electronic health records in U.S. hospitals. *New England Journal of Medicine* 360 (2009): 1628–1638.

Atwood, K. H pylori, plausibility, and Greek tragedy: The quirky case of Dr. John Lykoudis. *Science-Based Medicine: Exploring Issues and Controversies in the Relationship between Science and Medicine*, March 26, 2010. http://www.sciencebasedmedicine.org/?p=4238.

Balderjahn, I. Personality variables and environmental attitudes as predictors of ecologically responsible consumption patterns. *Journal of Business Research* 17 (1988): 51–56.

Begley, Sharon. The rush to biomarker tests. *Wall Street Journal*, December 12, 2006.

Behavior change theories and models. In *US Surgeon General's report on physical activity and health*, chapter 6, Understanding and promoting physical activity. http://www.csupomona.edu/~jvgrizzell/best_practices/bctheory .html.

Biomedicine: A vision for personalized medicine. *Technology Review*, March 9, 2010. http://www.technologyreview.com/biomedicine/24703/.

Bonner, T. N. *Iconoclast: Abraham Flexner and a life of learning.* Baltimore, MD: Johns Hopkins University Press, 2002.

Bremner, J. D. *Before you take that pill.* New York: Avery, 2008.

Carr, Nicholas. Is Google making us stupid? *The Atlantic* (July 2008).

Church, Dawson. Fighting the fire: Emotions, evolution and the future of psychology. *Energy Psychology Journal* (March 12, 2009): 1–7. http://energypsychologyjournal.org/?p=63.

Cloud, John. Why your DNA isn't your destiny. *Time,* January 6, 2010.

Connolly, P. H., V. J. Caiozzo, F. Zaldivar, D. Nemet, J. Larson, S. P. Hung, J. D. Heck, G. W. Hatfield, and D. M. Cooper. Effects of exercise on gene expression in human peripheral blood mononuclear cells. *Journal of Applied Physiology* 97 (2004): 1467–1469. doi: 10.1152/japplphysiol.00316.2004.

Cortese, D. A. A vision of individualized medicine in the context of global health. *Clinical Pharmacology & Therapeutics* 82 (2007): 491–493.

Davies, Kevin. Cracking the code of life: Nature vs. nurture revisited. April 17, 2001. http://www.pbs.org/wgbh/nova/genome/debate.html.

Dickler, H. B., et al. New physician-investigators receiving National Institutes of Health research project grants: a historical perspective on the "endangered species." *JAMA* 297 (2007): 2496.

Drug discovery. *Wikipedia.* http://en.wikipedia.org/wiki/Drug_discovery.

Ernst, E. A systematic review of systematic reviews of homeopathy. *British Journal of Clinical Pharmacology* 54 (2002): 577–582.

Ferry, G. Osler and after. *Oxford Today* 17, no. 3 (2005). http://www.oxfordtoday.ox.ac.uk/2004-05/v17n3/03.shtml.

Fischer, C. *Routine miracles: Personal journeys of patients and doctors discovering the power of modern medicine.* New York: Kaplan Publishing, 2009.

Friedman, E., M. Hayney, G. Love, H. Urry, M. Rosenkranz, R. Davidson, B. Singer, and C. Ryff. Social relationships, sleep quality, and interleukin-6 in aging women. *Proceedings of the National Academy of Sciences* 102 (2005): 18757–18762.

Friedman, Emily. Who should have access to your information: Privacy through the ethics lens. *Journal of AHIMA* 72 (2001): 24–27.

From education to regulation: Dynamic challenges to the health care workforce. Washington, DC: Association of Academic Health Centers (AAHC), 2008.

From the genome to the proteome. http://www.ornl.gov/sci/techresources /Human_Genome/project/info.shtml.

Gabbay, J., and A. Le May. *Practice-based evidence for healthcare.* London: Routledge Press, 2010.

Garfield, E. Essays of an information scientist: Creativity, delayed recognition, and other essays. *Current Contents* 12 (1989): 88–91.

Gleason, Bill. Why would an academic health center support homeopathy? *The Chronicle of Higher Education: Brainstorm*, January 22, 2011. http://chronicle.com/blogs/brainstorm/why-would-an-academic-health-center -support-homeopathy/31337.

Global antibiotics market to reach $40. 3 billion by 2015, according to new report by Global Industry Analysts, Inc. *PRWeb*, October 25, 2010. http://www.prweb.com/releases/antibiotics/anti_infectives/prweb4688824.htm.

Goetzel, R. Z., and R. J. Ozminkowski. The health cost benefits of work site health-promotion programs. *Annual Review of Public Health* 29 (2008): 303–323.

Goodwin, S. New Emory institute for drug discovery announced. (News release). May 19, 2009. http://whsc.emory.edu/home/news/releases/2009 /05/emory-institute-for-drug-discovery%20.

Health insurance costs: Facts on the cost of health insurance and health care. *National Coalition on Health Care* (August 2008). http://www.nchc.org /factsw/cost.shtml.

Heffern, R. Ecopsychology: Healthy planet, healthy people. *National Catholic Reporter*, December 28, 2010.

Holahan, C. Health social networking. *Bloomberg Businessweek,* June 16, 2008. http://businessweek.com/the_thread/techbeat/archives/2008/06 /health_social_network.

I get a kick out of you. *The Economist,* February 12, 2004.

International PPH Consortium, K. B. Lane, R. D. Machado, M. W. Pauciulo, J. R. Thomson, J. A. Phillips, J. E. Loyd, W. C. Nichols, and R. C. Trembath. Heterozygous germline mutations in BMPR2, encoding a TGF-beta receptor, cause familial primary pulmonary hypertension. *Nature Genetics* 26 (2000): 81–84.

Jeffrey P. Oh, take a pill. *Wall Street Journal,* August 1, 2008.

Johns, M., and K. Brigham. Transforming health care through prospective medicine: The first step. *Academic Medicine* 83 (2008): 706.

Johns, M. M. E. Pursuing Ponce's dream: Enabling the "square-wave life curve." *Medscape News,* September 15, 2006. http://www.medscape.com /viewarticle/543965.

Joint principles of the patient-centered medical home. American Academy of Family Physicians, American Academy of Pediatrics, American College of Physicians, American Osteopathic Association. March 2007. http://www.acponline.org/hpp/approve_jp.pdf.

Kilsheimer, Joe. Computers: Moderation is key to your cyberhealth. *Orlando Sentinel,* September 5, 1998.

Klein, S., N. F. Sjeard, X. Pi-Sunyer, A. Daly, J. Wylie-Rosett, K. Kulkarni, and N. G. Clark. Weight management through lifestyle modification for the prevention and management of type 2 diabetes: Rationale and strategies. (A statement of the American Diabetes Association, the North American Association for the Study of Obesity, and the American Society for Clinical Nutrition.) *American Journal of Clinical Nutrition* 80 (2004): 257–263.

Lambert, M. J., and G. M. Burlingame. Uniting practice-based evidence with evidence-based practice. *Behavioral Healthcare* (October 2007): 3.

Landro, Laura. Social networking comes to health care. *Wall Street Journal,* December 29, 2006.

Landro, Laura. *Survivor: Taking control of your fight against cancer.* New York: Simon & Schuster, 1998.

Lin, I. M., and E. Peper. Psychophysiological patterns during cell phone text messaging: a preliminary study. *Applied Psychophysiology and Biofeedback* 34 (2009): 53–57.

Lipton, Bruce. Maternal emotions and human development. *Birth Psychology* (n.d.). http://birthpsychology.com/free-article/maternal-emotions -and-human-development.

Marckmann, G., and K. W. Goodman. Introduction: Ethics of information technology in health care. *International Review of Information Ethics* 5 (2006): 2–5.

McGee, Tim. Monitor the environment through gene expression. http:// www.treehugger.com/files/2007/01/monitor_the_env.php.

McGlynn, E. A., S. M. Asch, J. Adams, J. Keesey, J. Hicks, A. DeCristoforo, and E. A. Kerr. The quality of health care delivered to adults in the United States. *New England Journal of Medicine* 348 (2003): 2635–2645.

Medical advances timeline. http://www.infoplease.com/ipa/A0932661.html.

Mendoza, E. R. Systems biology: Its past, present and potential. *Philippine Science Letters* 2 (2009): 16–34.

Nabel, Gary. The coordinates of truth. *Science* 326 (2009): 53–54.

New insights into human transcriptome revealed by deep sequencing study. http://www.medicalnewstoday.com/articles/114302.php.

Oliver, G., J. Wardle, and E. L. Gibson. Stress and food choice: A laboratory study. *Psychosomatic Medicine* 62 (2000): 853–865.

Pace, T., T. Mletzko, M. Alagbe, D. Musselman, C. Nemeroff, A. Miller, and C. Heim. Increased stress-induced inflammatory responses in male patients with major depression and increased early life stress. *American Journal of Psychiatry* 163 (2006): 1630–1633.

Paul, S. M., D. S. Mytelka, C. T. Dunwiddie, C. C. Persinger, B. H. Munos, S. R. Lindborg, and A. L. Schacht. How to improve R&D productivity: The pharmaceutical industry's grand challenge. *Nature Reviews Drug Discovery* 9 (2010): 203–214.

Pelletier, K. R. A review and analysis of the clinical and cost-effectiveness studies of comprehensive health promotion and disease management programs at the worksite: Update VII 2004–2008. *Journal of Occupational and Environmental Medicine* 51 (2009). doi: 10.1097/jom.0b013e3181 a7de5a.

Porter, M. E. What is value in health care? *New England Journal of Medicine* 363 (2010): 2477–2481.

Prochaska, J. O., and W. F. Velicer. The transtheoretical model of health behavior change. *American Journal of Health Promotion* 12 (1997): 38–48.

Robison, J. The business case for wellbeing. *Gallup Management Journal,* June 9, 2010, 1–7.

Rodriguez, K. *Nutritional genomics: Discovering the path to personalized nutrition.* New York: Wiley, 2006.

Schafer, A. I. Perspective: The successful physician-scientist of the 21st century. *CTSciNet,* May 28, 2010. http://sciencecareers.sciencemag.org/career _magazine/previous_issues/articles/2010_05_28/caredit.a1000054.

Schroeder, S. Jesuits, Nahuas, and the Good Death Society in Mexico City, 1710–1767. *Hispanic American Historical Review* 80, no. 1 (2000): 75.

Singer, B. H., and C. D. Ryff, eds. *New horizons in health: An integrative approach.* Washington, DC: National Academy Press, 2001.

Snyderman, R., and R. Williams. Prospective medicine: The next health care transformation. *Academic Medicine* 78 (2003): 79–84.

Snyderman, R., and Z. Yoediono. Perpective: Prospective health care and the role of academic medicine: Lead, follow or get out of the way. *Academic Medicine* 83 (1008): 707–714.

Sprenger, M. Issues at the interface of general practice and public health: Primary health care and our communities. *General Practice Online* (2005). http://priority.com/fam/gppublic.html.

Statin drugs (cholesterol fighters) and new side effects revealed? *Buzzle.com*, February 9, 2011. http://www.buzzle.com/articles/statin-drugs-cholesterol -fighters-and-new-side-effects-reveal.

Strecher, V. J., B. M. DeVellis, M. H. Becker, and I. M. Rosenstock. The role of self-efficacy in achieving health behavior change. *Health Education Quarterly* 13 (1986): 73–91.

Studies on nutrients, gene expression could lead to tailored diets for disease prevention. http://www.eurekalert.org/pub_releases/2010–03/ksu-son03 0510.php.

Sui, X., M. J. LaMonte, J. N. Laditka, et al. Cardiorespiratory fitness and adiposity as mortality predictors in older adults. *JAMA* 298 (2007): 2507–2516.

The Galileo Project. http://galileo.rice.edu/bio/narrative_7.html.

The health of nations. *The Economist,* July 17, 2004.

Twiss, S. B. The problem of moral responsibility in medicine. *Journal of Medicine and Philosophy* 2 (1977): 330–375.

UK Biobank. http://www.mrc.ac.uk/Ourresearch/Ethicsresearchguidance /Biobank/index.htm.

Voit, E. O., and K. L. Brigham. The role of systems biology in predictive health and personalized medicine. *The Open Pathology Journal* 2 (2008): 68–70.

Wagner, J. The future of nutraceuticals. *Nutritional Outlook* (June/July 2002). http://www.fimdefelice.org/clippings/clip.future.html.

Walker, W. A., and G. Blackburn. Symposium introduction: Nutrition and gene regulation. *Journal of Nutrition* 134 (2004): 2434s–2436s.

Welch, H. G., L. M. Schwartz, and S. Woloshin. *Overdiagnosed: Making people sick in the pursuit of health*. Boston: Beacon Press, 2011.

What is a patient centered medical home? An overview to patient centered medical homes for patients from the Patient Centered Primary Care Collaborative. http://www.pcpcc.net/content/pcmh-videos.

Wolever, R. Q., M. Dreusicke, J. Fikkan, T. V. Hawkins, S. Yeung, J. Wakefield, L. Duda, P. Flowers, C. Cook, and E. Skinner. Integrative health coaching for patients with type 2 diabetes: A randomized clinical trial. *Diabetes Education* 36 (2010): 629–639.

Zeidner, M., and M. Schechter. Psychological responses to air pollution: some personality and demographic correlates. *Journal of Environmental Psychology* 8 (1988): 191–208.

Zellner, D. A., S. Loaiza, Z. Gonzalez, J. Pita, J. Morles, D. Pecora, and A. Wolf. Food selection changes under stress. *Physiology & Behavior* 7 (2006): 789–793.

Zemlo, T. R., H. H. Garrison, N. C. Partridge, and T. J. Ley. The physician-scientist: career issues and challenges at the year 2000. *FASEB Journal* 14, no. 2 (2000): 221–230.

Index